SIMPLE MEDICINE

3 MINUTES MANAGEMENT

(SM- 3MM)

Part 1

2020

Lt Col (R) Dr Zuki Othman

Contents

1. Disclaimer — -3

2. Prologue — -4

3. **Chapter 1**: Medical Screening I — -8

4. **Chapter 2**: Medical Screening II — -29

5. **Chapter 3**: Making Sense of the Medical Treatment — -40

6. **Chapter 4**: Iatrogenic Problems — -50

7. **Chapter 5**: The Choosing Wisely Project — -57

8. **Chapter 6**: The Common Complaints and Treatment:
    A.   Back-Pain — -63

9. **Chapter 7**: The Common Complaints and Treatment:
    B.   Headaches, Migraines, Dizzy Spells & Fainting
    Attacks — -82

10. **Chapter 8**: The Common Complaints and Treatment:
    C.   Upper Respiratory Tract Infections (URTIs)
    - Common Cold and Flu — -101

11. **Chapter 9**: Covid-19 and Other Infectious Diseases — -125

12. **Chapter 10**: Treatment for Kids — -139

13. **Chapter 11**: Government Hospitals vs. Private Hospitals — -151

14. **Chapter 12**: SM- 3MM — -168

Disclaimer

"The information provided in this book is designed to provide helpful information on the subjects discussed. This book is not meant to be used, nor should it be used, to diagnose or treat any medical conditions. For diagnosis or treatment of any medical problems, consult your physician.

The publisher and author are not responsible for any specific health or allergy needs that may require medical supervision and are not liable for any damages or negative consequences from any treatment, action, application or preparation, to any person reading or following the information in this book.

References are provided for informational purposes only and do not constitute endorsement of any websites or other sources. Readers should be aware that the websites listed in this book may change".

Dr Zuki Othman

<u>PROLOGUE</u>

TANGIER, MOROCCO.
JULY 2018

'There are no foreign lands. It is the traveller who is foreign'.
-    Robert Louis Stevenson

"Why don't you write a book about that?" asked my wife. "I will", I replied. "I will start writing the book once I have been to Tangier", I continued.

What did I complain to my wife? Well, since I resigned from the Malaysian Armed Forces Health Services (MAFHS) in 2009 I had been complaining to my wife that how surprised I was with the very different ways of treating the patients in the **private sectors** as compared to the military services or to the government hospitals .

Both are not wrong, like getting loans from the banks. And we have so many big and efficient banks in Malaysia. But too many loans would make your life very miserable, and some people would even end up committing suicide because of having too much loans that overwhelm their abilities to repay them.

It is the same with the medical screening and medical treatment. You should not just simply be doing most or all of the medical screening that are available on the market, or go for the medical treatment for every simple medical problems that you have.

Once I had a young lady in her 20s from one of the western countries requesting for blood tests. She wanted to do all these tests because her **homeopathic doctor** asked her to do them. She handed to me a piece of paper that listed all the tests that she wanted to do and she wanted to do them urgently.

The tests that she wanted to do were the Cholesterol Profiles, the Thyroid Hormones, the Female Hormones, all the Tumour Marker tests including the Epstein Barr Virus Antibodies, Fasting Blood Sugar and HbA1c for Diabetes, the Ferritin level, the Homocystein test, the Cortisol level and a few other tests that I did not understand.

These were a lot of tests for a young lady without any medical problems. We did not do any of these tests for our young female fighter pilots when I was in the Royal Malaysian Air-Force before.

Why did I mention Tangier in my answer to my wife above? Why not other famous cities in the world? There were a few reasons for me to keep mentioning Tangier as **an excuse not to write this book.**

The first reason was that Tangier to me symbolised a charmed, rustic and mysterious old city. This city has seen many civilisations and cultures for the past few thousand years. This is the city where Ibn Battuta, the greatest explorer of all time was born on the 24th of February 1304.

In June 1325 at the age of 21, he started his journey. Initially he travelled to Mecca for his pilgrimage. He then continued his journey to most of the countries that existed at that time in North Africa, the Horn of Africa, West Africa, the Middle East, Central Asia, South-East Asia, South Asia and China.

He did not return to Tangier for the next 24 years. When he did go back, he continued his journey for another 6 years to Europe and North African countries. In those 30 years of travelling, he covered about 117,000 km of distance.

This was about twice the distance as covered by Marco Polo, another great world traveller and explorer. One of the similarities between these two great explorers is that they started their journeys at a very young age, 17 for Marco Polo and 21 for Ibn Battuta.

Can you imagine my dismay when I had so many young patients who regularly complained of various simple medical problems at my clinics? These problems included frequent headaches, migraines, dizzy spells, fainting attacks, neck pain, back pain, stomach pain, heart-burns, bodyache, tiredness and many more. Some even complained of having low immunity levels, which is very ridiculous.

If they complain of these symptoms at the government clinics, they would have been treated with simple medication. Since they came to the private clinics, we needed to do something with their complaints. **Most people believe that doing more tests or seeing more specialists are better** (which is not true).

Many of them would request for referrals to the private specialists such as the gastro-enterologists, the neurologists, the neurosurgeons, the ENT surgeons, the orthopaedic surgeons, the gynaecologists, the obstetricians or the psychiatrists. Some of them would even be admitted to the hospitals for more investigations or treatment.

During those specialist's appointments or hospital admissions, they would have been thoroughly investigated with full blood and urine tests, x-rays, ultra-sounds, or even with the MRIs and CT scans. In most cases, the results were normal or insignificant. Yet they were very puzzled that the doctors did not or could not find anything wrong with them.

Because of these complaints, most of them spent so much of their precious time on medical leaves, on appointments or on hospital admissions. Sometimes they even went for invasive procedures or operations.

For me young people should be happy, optimistic, positive, energetic, they should go travelling, live their lives to the fullest, work hard, further their studies or they may try to change the world. They are not supposed to be worried about simple medical problems, unnecessary medical investigations or hospital admissions.

The second and more important reason why I mentioned Tangier above was because I thought that I would never have the opportunities to visit Tangier in my whole life. I might have gone to Tangier easily if I were still a student, or single, or if I were still in the military, but not at this time, when I had a young family to look after and a few private clinics to take care of.

However, here I was, in the late July 2018, walking along the Mohammed VI Avenue towards the new Tangier Marina Bay. The new Bay is a massive new redevelopment of the Port of Tangier Ville to cater to cruise ships and yachts. They hope that one day the city would become a leading tourist destination. Unfortunately, now most tourists would just bypass Tangier and go to other cities like Marrakesh, Casablanca or Agadir.

The Port of Tangier Ville is located in the western part of the city, at the entrance of the Straits of Gibraltar, which is situated on a bay between Cap Spartel and Cap Malabata. When I googled the map it was breath-taking to see that we were on top of the African Continent, on the western side and was very close to Southern Europe.

Since I have been to Tangier, now I have to keep the promise that I made to my wife. Yes, a promise is a promise. Now I have to start writing the book that I never plan to write or had any intentions of writing.

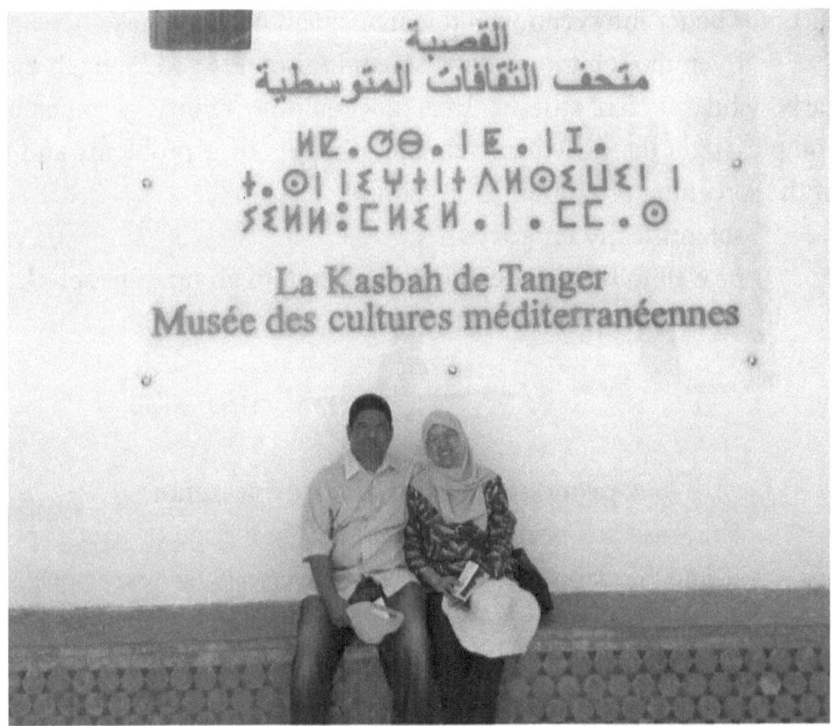

Picture-1: La Kasbah de Tanger: July, 2018.

CHAPTER 1

MEDICAL SCREENING I

'After you find out all the things that can go wrong, your life becomes less about living and more about waiting'.

- *Chuck Palahniuk, Choke*

What is a Medical Screening? ***'A Medical screening is the systematic application of a series of test or inquiry that we do in a normal, healthy people with no medical problems and without having any signs or symptoms to identify the possible presence of an as-yet-undiagnosed disease'***. Its purpose is to identify the disease early for better intervention and management of the disease.

Even though the medical screening sounds good - catch disease early while it can still be treated - but the reality is much more complex than that. Medical screening has its own problems and most of the screening programmes are either:

1. scientifically unproven.
2. proven to be beneficial only in a certain group of people.
3. could be harmful in the long run.

<u>Case No. 1</u>
Tan Sri A,
A prominent Malaysian Businessman.

This case has been widely reported in the major newspapers in Malaysia and Singapore for the past 15 years. The reason we knew about this case is that it involved a very prominent businessman, and a Tan Sri on top of that. I am sure that there were many other cases like his, but since the patients were not well known, then we will never knew about them. (*Sources- Google: 'A prominent Malaysian businessman sued a Singapore hospital'*).

I want to stress here that who this businessman is, is not important. However, his case is very essential for us to learn about the possible complications arising from doing a simple medical check-up.

It was reported that everything started in 2003 when he was found to have a nodule in his right lung from his chest x-ray. Since you won't have any symptoms from a lung nodule, I presumed that he went for a full medical check-up. It is very common in Malaysia for people who are above 40 years old (some are even much younger) to go for a full medical check-up.

By the middle of 2010, this nodule was found to have grown from about 12mm to 18mm in diameter. The doctors in Malaysia thought that this was a Neuro-Endocrine Tumour ('NET') of low-grade malignancy.

They referred him to one of the leading cancer hospitals in Singapore to undergo a Positron Emission Tomography (PET) scan using a radioisotope Gallium 68 tagged with Dotatate (the Gallium Scan). This PET scan was done with a Computed Tomography-Scan (CT-Scan), which together they were called 'The Gallium PET/CT Scan'.

The Gallium PET/CT Scan is supposed to be the ***gold standard*** test for the NETs. In other words, the test can confirm whether the patient has the NETs or not. As an ex- military doctor and a doctor that used to be involved in the medical check-ups of our Royal Malaysian Air Force pilots and in the Malaysian Astronaut Programme candidates, routine medical examinations can be very misleading.

Therefore, we did not look at the minor, insignificant abnormalities, instead we looked at the general and overall results of the medical tests and the conditions of the person. For example if you have many abnormal readings in your blood tests, we just ignore them unless the abnormal values are significant, or something else is significant.

From all these tests, the doctors were even more convinced that he had the NETs, which would affect his endocrine glands. The endocrine glands can be found in many organs such as in the pancreas, adrenal glands and testes. The doctors concluded that he might have a tumour in his pancreas or a ***pancreatic tumour.***

He was then advised to go for a major operation by the Singapore Surgical Oncologist to remove his pancreatic tumour. The operation which was done in August 2010 was a complex and difficult one, where the doctors removed part of his five organs. These five organs were the head of the pancreas, the first part of the small intestine (duodenum), the gallbladder, the bile duct and part of the stomach.

He developed severe complications from the operation and nearly died due to that complications. He had to go for two other operations to repair the complications arising from the first operation. What made him angry was when he found out from the **Laboratory Reports** that all the organs removed including the head of the pancreas were normal. It meant that he did not have any tumour at all. He was in fact healthy, and did not have to go for any of the operations in the first place.

Now he claims that he could not be active physically due to the complications from the operations. He also has problems in eating since the doctors had removed part of his stomach, duodenum, gall bladder, the bile duct as well as the pancreas. Therefore, he sued the doctor and the hospital for medical error, but he lost. He appealed the verdict in **2016**, but also lost the case.

I do not want to go into details about his litigation, but we can learn a few things from this case:

1. A simple medical check-up or a chest x-ray could lead to three unnecessary operations.

2. Even a prominent consultant at one of the leading hospitals in Singapore could be led to do unnecessary operations due to misleading test results.

3. Expensive tests such as the MRIs, CT scans and even the Gallium PET/CT Scan, which was supposed to be the gold standard test or a diagnostic test as in the case above can lead to a wrong diagnosis.

4.   A person who was perfectly normal without any complaints, who went for a medical check-up could end up worse than before the medical check-up.

<u>Case No. 2</u>
Mr AB,
A Malaysian Lawyer.

Mr AB went for a regular medical check-up or a medical screening in India. He was found to have **a possible cyst** on his left kidney. After coming back to Malaysia he went to a private hospital on 11 Nov 2014 for a further management of his problem. At this hospital he was told that his problem was not a left renal cyst, but **a left kidney cancer** or **a left renal cell carcinoma**. *(Source: Google- 3 hospitals, 8 doctors face RM45 million suit over wrong diagnosis).*

He went to another 2 hospitals for a second and a third opinion, and these two hospitals gave him the same diagnosis. He claimed that he was advised to go for **an urgent operation** to remove his left kidney to prevent the cancerous cells from spreading to other organs.

However, he sought a fourth opinion by a nephrologist at another hospital and found that there was **no cancer** on his left kidney. Both of his kidneys were perfectly normal. Now he is suing the first 3 hospitals and demanding over RM45 million in damages from the hospitals in 3 separate negligence suits against them and eight doctors who treated him.

He claimed that he had to spend a lot of money to pay for the CT scans, biopsies, ultrasounds and other tests and treatments, all of which also took up a lot of his time.

Again, I am not going to discuss about his court cases here. But we can see how a simple routine medical check-up could end up with more and more tests being done including the ultrasounds, CT-scans and the kidney biopsies. He was also given with **3 very different diagnoses**, first with a possible left kidney cyst, second with a left kidney cancer by 3 different hospitals and finally with a normal kidney.

<u>**Litigation Against Doctors**</u>

Before I continue further, I would like to write a few things about litigation against doctors. Nowadays in Malaysia we see more and more of litigation cases brought upon doctors by the patients. Even though we need a law to protect and enforce the rights of the patients and to solve conflicts, but this court process can be **a double-edged sword.**

Suing doctors will make more and more doctors practicing **defensive medicine,** not the **best practice medicine.** Defensive medicine is a practice of doing excessive diagnostic testing or excessive medical treatment that is not necessarily the best option for the patient, but mainly serves to protect the doctor against the patient as potential litigant.

Defensive medicine is also a reaction to the rising costs of malpractice insurance premiums and patients' biases on suing for mistreatment. Some of the doctors would avoid treating high-risk patients (when they have a choice) to reduce their exposure to lawsuits, or are forced to discontinue practicing because of overly high insurance premiums.

They will also make the cost of the treatment in the future much more expensive as the doctors need to pay more for the medical insurance premium rates, to pay for more tests as to make sure that the diagnosis is 100 percent accurate, to pay higher fee to more specialised doctors to do even a simple procedure etc.

<u>**The Problems With The Medical Screening**</u>

As you can see from the above cases, even expensive tests such as the MRIs, CT-scans and even the Gallium-PET/CT Scan, which is supposed to be the gold standard test for the Neuro-Endocrine Tumour (NET) can lead to a wrong conclusion or diagnosis.

Medical Screening can become harmful for example by having **False Positive Results,** as in the cases above**,** where a doctor sees a lesion that looks like a cancer but it is not. These false positive results would lead to other unnecessary, expensive and sometimes dangerous additional tests, procedures or treatment.

Medical Screening can also lead to over-diagnosis and over-treatment. An **Over-diagnosis** is when doctors find a problem for e.g. a cancer that would not have gone on to cause any symptoms or problems, or may even go away on its own. Treatment of these cancer is called an **over-treatment**. These over-treatment can cause unnecessary and unwanted side effects.

Another problem with the medical screening is the **False Negative Results**, where the tests miss the problems e.g. miss a cancer, which may delay finding that cancer and getting the appropriate treatment.

Basically, Medical Screening divides the people into two categories, those who are likely and those who are unlikely to develop the problem. ***Unfortunately, for screening to be effective in a general population, large numbers of healthy people would have to be tested***. Usually, some of them will be found to have some sort of abnormalities, which are not significant but could lead to further tests to confirm that these abnormalities are 100% normal.

The medical test used for the screening purposes are often not suitable in making a final diagnosis. Instead, the screening tests are used to detect for abnormalities first, which then require more tests to be done to look at these abnormalities more closely.

There are doubts whether many of the routine medical screening are advantageous or not, but during the last decade they have increased in popularity not only in the developed countries but also in the developing countries.

In Malaysia, medical screening has become a big business. It has become something like routine tests that people need to do every year or do it regularly. Now every clinic, hospital and even a pharmacy and a medical laboratory is doing the screening tests.

Medical Screening does not set a 'gold standard' as an examination method. There is no ideal screening method that has been discovered yet. **Therefore, a healthy life style is much more important regarding health in general, which screening cannot replace.**

A. <u>MAMMOGRAM TEST FOR BREAST CANCER</u>

Since Breast Cancer is the number one cancer among women in Malaysia and also in the whole world, and mammogram is one of the most common screening tests for the Breast Cancer, I would use the mammogram test as an example of the complex nature of a medical screening programme.

A mammogram is done by taking x-ray images and using them to examine the breast for the early detection of cancer and also for detecting other breast diseases. Therefore, it is used as both a **diagnostic** and a **screening** tool.

In Breast Cancer screening, the mammograms usually will find lesions of uncertain significance- cancer that do not behave aggressively. *Since we do not usually have the ability to work out which of these cancer will spread and cause death, most women with abnormal results are offered treatment, which include a mastectomy operation, a radiation therapy and a chemotherapy.*

These treatment can do harm. For example, surgery comes with the usual risks from the surgery itself, from the anaesthetic and from the potential for infection, radiotherapy slightly raises the risk of later heart disease and chemotherapy has many side effects such as nausea, vomiting, loss of appetite, fatigue and hair loss.

These risks may well be worth taking if the breast disease threatens your life, but it is far less clear what to do when the screening has picked up a potentially **harmless lesion**.

1. <u>The Problems with Mammograms in the UK and Sweden</u>
Professor Dr Michael Baum was a Professor Emeritus of surgery at the University College London and a consultant in the Surgical Oncologist. In 1988, he was one of the doctors that set up the service for the **UK NHS Breast Screening Programme (NHSBSP)**. More than 20 years later, **he has called for the programme to be shut down**, arguing it leads to healthy women being labeled 'cancer victims' and has not reduced the number of invasive tumours.
(Sources- Google: "Dr Michael Baum, mammogram, should be scrapped').

He estimated that 10,000 women would need to be screened with mammograms to prevent 3-4 deaths (which means that the benefit is very small)**, but this screening test would lead to 120-140 normal women being over-diagnosed,** and having unnecessary treatment.

Again, an **Over-diagnosis** here refers to the detection of cancer on screening, which **would not have become clinically apparent in the woman's lifetime** in the absence of the screening, or this is where the **non-growing or slow-growing, harmless cancer** are found.

These women would have led to a normal life without the need to go for the Breast Cancer treatment if they have not gone for the mammogram screening program.

Referring to the statistics in Table-1 below, according to Prof. Dr Michael Baum, for every 10,000 women screened with mammograms, they manage to save 3-4 lives. Unfortunately since the mammogram test is not accurate, at the same time they **would over-diagnose between 120-140 healthy women**, who would end-up with the same treatment as the women with the Breast Cancer would get even though they do not have any significant Breast Cancer.

	MAMMOGRAM TEST		
SER	**NO OF WOMEN TESTED**	**NO OF LIVES SAVED**	**NO. OF WOMEN <u>OVER-DIAGNOSED</u> WITH CANCER**
1.	10,000	3 - 4	120 - 140
2.	2,000,000 (No. Of Tests in the UK Per Year)	600 - 800	*24,000 - 28,000*

Table-1: The Outcome of the Mammogram Tests in the UK according to Prof. Dr. Michael Baum.

Since they are doing about 2,000,000 mammogram tests every year in the UK, they would have saved between 600 - 800 lives, but at the same time they would **over-diagnose between 24,000 - 28,000 normal women** that would be labeled as having Breast Cancer.

'Back in 1988, in all good faith, I set up the service for the NHS Breast Screening Programme (NHSBHP). **Since then, I have become one of the most vociferous proponents for closing it down,'** said Prof. Dr Michael Baum in **2016** in *The Hippocratic Post*. 'You probably want to know why I changed my mind so completely. *(Source:Refer:https://www.hippocraticpost.com/cancer/screening-breast-cancer-short- history-big-mistake/)*

'At the heart of this is the question, how do you explain to a woman that she is 'lucky' that we caught her Breast Cancer early yet she ends up having a mastectomy? And that she probably wouldn't have needed treatment at all if we hadn't called her in for a routine scan?' He continued.

One of the reasons for this is because mammograms can pick up a type of low-grade Breast Cancer called 'Duct Carcinoma In Situ' (DCIS), which is contained just in the milk ducts and has not spread into any of the surrounding breast tissue. Around half of these cancer turn out to be harmless. He thought that too many healthy women were harmed by the Breast Cancer screening.

A separate study found women were more likely to have **over-diagnosed Breast Cancer than early detection of a tumour** destined to grow significantly if they do the mammogram tests. Any reduction in the Breast Cancer deaths, researchers said was **due to the treatment, not screening**. *(Source: Breast-Cancer Tumor Size, Overdiagnosis, and Mammography Screening Effectiveness,* **October 13, 2016***, N Engl J Med 2016; 375:1438-1447)*

All women in England diagnosed early with the mammograms are treated comprehensively, even though some have over-diagnosed, harmless cancer. These women cannot benefit from the treatment but are exposed to the physical, psychological and social harm of the cancer treatment.

In another review also raised the disturbing possibility that **mammogram screening could be doing more harm than good**. *(Source: Cochrane Systematic Review -'Screening for Breast Cancer with mammography')*. Its authors said: 'This means that **for every 2,000 women invited for screening throughout the 10 years period, one will have her life prolonged,** and **10 healthy women, who would not have been diagnosed if there had not been screening, will be diagnosed as Breast Cancer patients** and **will be treated**

unnecessarily. Furthermore, **more than 200 other women** will experience unnecessary psychological distress for many months because of the **false positive findings** with more and more tests being done until they are confirmed to be normal.

Professor Dr Peter Gøtzsche, the co-founder of the independent Nordic Cochrane Collaboration, has spent more than 15 years investigating and analysing data from the trials of the breast screening that were run mostly in Sweden, before countries such as the UK introduced their national programme. He is a Danish Physician, medical researcher and former leader of the Nordic Cochrane Center in Coppenhagen, Denmark.

In his book '**Mammography Screening: Truth, Lies and Controversy**', which was originally published in **2012**, stated that **Breast Cancer screening can no longer be justified**, because **the harm to many women from needless diagnosis and damaging treatment outweighs the small number of lives saved.**
(Source: Google- 'Mammography screening: truth, lies and controversy').

The data that Prof. Dr Gøtzsche maintained for more than a decade does not support mass screening as a preventive measure. He said: 'Screening does not cut Breast Cancer deaths by 30% as commonly believed. **It saves probably one life for every 2,000 women who go for the mammogram. But it harms 10 others**'.

'Cancerous cells that will go away or never progress to disease in the woman's lifetime are excised with surgery and sometimes (six times in 10) she will lose a breast. Treatment with radiotherapy, chemotherapy and other drugs, as well as the surgery itself, all have a heavy mental and physical cost', he continued.

Case No. 3
Dr IP,
A Breast Surgeon, UK.

Dr IP is a very respected breast surgeon in the UK. In **2017** he was found guilty of over-diagnosing and over-treating thousands of patients with Breast Cancer during his career as a Breast Surgeon between **1997 and 2011 with unnecessary operations**.

(Source: Google- UK breast surgeon found guilty for unnecessary operations).

He was initially sentenced to 15 years in prison, but later increased to 20 years to demonstrate the seriousness of his offence. There were many things that he did wrong, but I am sure that suspicious mammogram results were one of the reasons why so many women went to him for further management of their problems.

Since he was found guilty, the UK NHS and Spire Health Care, the hospital group where Paterson treated his private patients have paid £37.2m of compensation (as in September 2017) to about 1,000 of his patients. There are thousands more patients that could sue him and the NHS.

2.   <u>The Problems with Mammograms in Malaysia</u>

It is the same problem in Malaysia. Our incidence rate for Breast Cancer in Malaysia is lower than in the UK, about 4,500 – 5,000 new cases per year. Therefore, we would have the Incidence Rate of 2 new cases of Breast Cancer for every 1,000 adult woman every year. (*Incidence Rate = the number of new breast cancer every year divide by the total number of Adult Women in Malaysia*).

If 1,000 women in Malaysia randomly do the mammogram tests, the best result that we could get is to pick up those two new cases of Breast Cancer. Yes, at best, the mammogram tests could only pick up two cases of new Breast Cancer patients for every 1,000 Malaysian women tested.

There are a few terms that we should know when we are talking about the medical screening. A Sensitive test or **Sensitivity** means that the test is able to correctly identify those with the disease, to give the **True Positive Rate**. A Specific test or **Specificity** is the ability of that test to correctly identify those without the disease, to give the **True Negative Rate**.

Since the **Sensitivity** of the mammogram test would never be 100% accurate, we would never pick up that two new cases of the

Breast Cancer in the Malaysian Population. What we would pick up is less than that and at the same time, since the **Specificity of the mammogram test** would also never be 100% **accurate,** we would wrongly diagnose other healthy women who actually do not have a cancer with a Breast Cancer.

Another important thing to remember here is that, since the nature of the medical screening is **to detect a small number of positive cases in a large number of healthy population**, even a slight decrease in the Specificity of the test will make us to over-diagnose a large number of healthy women. For e.g. if the Specificity of the mammogram test here is 95% accurate, we would over-diagnose 50 normal women that do not have a Breast Cancer with a Breast Cancer for every 1,000 women screened with the mammograms.

Whereas for the Sensitivity of the test, even if the sensitivity of the mammogram test is 100% accurate, since statistically there would only be 2 possible Breast Cancer for every 1,000 women in Malaysia, we would only pick up 2 cases of new Breast Cancer for every 1,000 women that go for the mammogram test.

The Formula how to get the rate of the Sensitivity and Specificity are shown in Table- 2 below.

a.   <u>Defining Sensitivity and Specificity</u>

SER	CONDITION TEST RESULTS	Condition Present	Condition Absent
1.	Positive Result	True Positive (A)	False Positive (B)
2.	Negative Result	False Negative (C)	True Negative (D)

Table-2: Defining Sensitivity and Specificity.
A. Sensitivity = A / (A+C), b. Specificity = D / (B+D)

Even without doing the mammogram tests, we could still be able to detect those 2 new cases of Breast Cancer for every 1,000 women every year by using other methods, such as the breast examination (either self-examination or examined by a doctor), CT-scans, Ultra-sounds or Breast Biopsies.

b.   <u>Results of The Mammogram Tests in Malaysia</u>

According to one of the professors from a leading medical school in Malaysia, for every 1,000 random adult women in Malaysia that go for the mammogram tests, the results would be as shown in Table-3 below.

SER	TEST TYPE	MAMMOGRAM TESTS		
		NO OF WOMEN TESTED	RESULTS	
			NORMAL	SUSPICIOUS
1.	Random	1,000	900	100
2.	Further Tests	100	60	40
Nb: Only 2 out of 1,000 women would have Breast Cancer every year				

Table-3. The Mammogram Results in Malaysia.

We would have 100 suspicious results (98 of them with normal breasts and 2 with possible Breast Cancer) for every 1,000 women tested randomly with the mammograms in Malaysia. These 100 women with suspicious results would be asked to go for further tests such as additional mammograms, ultrasound tests, MRI scans or breast biopsies.

Most of the time these 100 women with suspicious results would be continuously worrying about their suspicious results and would continue asking for further tests. Usually some of them would seek a second or a third opinion at other hospitals and some would even end up with operations even though they do not really have the Breast Cancer (as what happened in Case No. 3 above).

So, at best, the mammogram tests in Malaysia could only pick up 2 new Breast Cancer patients for every 1,000 women tested. But at worst it could over-diagnose between 38 to 98 normal women with Breast Cancer.

<u>Case No. 4</u>
Ms F, A 50 y.o Lady.

In 2009 Ms F complained of having pain and discomfort in both of her breasts. She also felt that she was having a breast lump in her left breast. She went to see one of the Breast Surgeons at a private hospital in the Klang Valley. She was advised to go for an urgent mammogram test.

According to her, the results of the mammogram test showed that she had a Stage 3 Breast Cancer measuring 10.3 cm in her left breast and 0.7 cm in her right breast. She was then advised to go for an emergency operation to remove both cancers from her breasts.

However, she did not agree with the operations and requested for a discharge from the hospital. She decided not to do anything with her problems. I met her in 2020 and she had no problems with her breasts anymore. The pain and the lump that she felt in her breasts 11 years ago had disappeared a few months later and now she does not feel any lumps in her breasts.

I was shocked to hear that and did not know how to advice her. I presumed that the cancer that the doctors detected in 2009 could be one of the false positive results that they got from the mammogram test. If the diagnosis were correct, she should have been dead by now or her cancer should have spread all over her body.

B.   <u>**PAP SMEAR TESTS FOR CERVICAL CANCER**</u>

It is the same issue with a pap smear, another common screening procedure for Cervical Cancer. The Cervical Cancer is the second or third most common cancer among women in Malaysia (according to the year) after the Breast Cancer.

Pap Smear is a procedure in which a small brush or spatula is used to gently remove cells from the cervix through a vagina so that they can be **checked under a microscope** for Cervical Cancer cells or cell changes that may lead to Cervical Cancer.

But most cervical-cell changes found at a pap smear screening will not lead to Cervical Cancer. The problem is we can't predict which will, so all need further monitoring or treatment.

A study from Bristol, UK in **2003** came to the following conclusions: (*Refer: BMJ.2003 Apr 26; 326(7395):901 'Outcomes of* *screening to prevent cancer: analysis of cumulative incidence of cervical abnormality and modelling of cases and deaths prevented'*).

1.   In the NHS, UK cervical screening programme, ***around 1,000 women would need to be screened for 35 years to prevent one death from Cervical Cancer*** (which means that the benefit is very small).

2.   Over 80% of women with high grade Cervical Intra-epithelial Neoplasia (CIN) will not develop invasive cancer, but all need to be either further investigated or treated.

3.   ***For each death prevented, over 150 women have an abnormal results, over 80 are referred for investigations, and over 50 have treatment even though they do not have the Cervical Cancer.***

4.   Before the 1988 relaunch of screening with strict quality standard, for each death prevented there were 57,000 tests and 1,955 women had abnormal results (the tests were less accurate before).

From the conclusions above, they found that they only saved 1 life in every 35 years for every 1,000 women that went for the pap smear tests. But at the same time they would have had 150 abnormal results, with 80 of them were referred for further tests, and 50 of them would end up with the same treatment as the one diagnosed with Cervical Cancer, even though they did not have any significant cancer cells.

Since the number of Cervical Cancer cases in Malaysia is less than the Breast Cancer, about 2,000 to 3,000 cases per year, and the results from the Pap Smears are more operator dependant, then there are more suspicious results in the Pap Smear tests compared to the mammogram tests.

If we do 1,000 pap smear tests randomly in Malaysia, at best we could only detect 1 new Cervical Cancer case. (The Incidence Rate of the Cervical Cancer in Malaysia is only 1 in 1,000. *The Incidence Rate = The Number of New Cases Every Year/ The Number of Adult women*).

Unfortunately, since the pap smear test is not accurate, we would over-diagnose hundreds of normal women with abnormal findings or even with cancer, even though they do not have any significant cancer cells in their cervix for every 1,000 women tested.

These suspicious results would then lead to other unnecessary tests, procedures or even operations.

C. <u>PROSTATE-SPECIFIC ANTIGEN (PSA) TEST.</u>

The problems of the Breast Cancer and Cervical Cancer **over-diagnoses** are similar to the problems faced by men diagnosed with Prostate Cancer using a **Prostate-Specific Antigen (PSA)** blood test. **These men have a cancer that is so slow growing that it would have never been detected otherwise.**

That is why the U.S. Preventive Services Task Force in **2013** has proposed that the routine PSA screening to be abandoned. The task force says that most men whose Prostate Cancer were detected through screening **are over-diagnosed**.

One of the reasons why PSA screening is very controversial is that an abnormal PSA test does not always mean that the Prostate Cancer is present. In addition, men with a normal PSA test can still have the Prostate Cancer. There are many reasons for this variation, one of them is the prostate size. Men with enlarged prostate glands would produce more PSA even though they are normal.

Therefore, they recommend that the annual PSA tests might be beneficial only for men over 45 with family histories of Prostate Cancer. ***For men with no family history of Prostate Cancer, the test is not beneficial at all.***

The American Urological Association (AUA) has released new guidelines in 2013 regarding PSA testing which are:

(Refer:1. Google: AUA new clinical guidelines on PSA or go to 2. http://auanet.mediaroom.com/2013-05-03-Aua-Releases-New-Clinical-Guideline-On-Prostate-Cancerscreening?articleNo=290)

1. Men under 40 should not do PSA tests.
2. Men ages 40 to 50 **should not be tested, if they are at average risk for the disease.** Those at **higher risk**- such as African-American men and those with a family history of Prostate Cancer- *should talk it over with their doctors first* (a polite way of saying that not 100% of these men need to do the tests)

3.   **For men 55 to 69, the test makes the most sense**. The AUA panel recommends *a shared decision by doctors and patients about the test*. Once testing begins, the panel says it should be done every two years, rather than annually.

4.   Men over 70 and with less than a 10 to 15 years life expectancy can probably skip the test.

'The Popularity Paradox'

Since most of the screening tests and the treatment at the private clinics and hospitals in Malaysia are either paid by the employers or they are cheap if compared to other countries, many people would happily do them without even considering whether they want to take the **risks for the potential harms** caused by such tests or treatment.

As the medical screening is not that accurate as explained above, these patients that go for the medical screening may not know if their screening tests would cause them harm from having the unnecessary procedures, treatment or surgeries.

This leads to the "popularity paradox" where a bad screening test creates many false positives results (to wrongly diagnose those without a disease as having a disease) as in the Cases No.1, 2, 3 and 4 above, which then lead to many unnecessary procedures, treatment and even surgeries, but people end up feeling that they "owe their life" to the screening tests.

However, in reality, they have been subjected to the unnecessary procedures, treatment and surgeries, and to the risks due to all of them.

Human Errors In Other Systems

Some of my patients asked why these errors could happen in the medical system. Actually similar errors could happen in every system that we have in this world, as happen in the cases below. Some of them cause much more damages to the human lives and properties as well as the monetary losses than compared to the cost of medical errors in the medical system.

<u>Case No. 5</u>
Mr AW,
America's Got Talent (AGT) 2020 Contestant,
The Judicial System.

In 1982, a 30 years old white woman in Louisiana, USA was raped and stabbed in her home. Luckily she survived the ordeal. Mr AW, a black guy was caught and brought to court. He denied of committing the crime as he was sleeping at his house during that time. He had 3 people that confirmed the story. Furthermore, none of the fingerprints found at the crime scene matched his fingerprints. *(Source: Google- America's 2020 Got Talent contestant wrongfully convicted).*

But the state wanted somebody to pay for the crime. In 1983 he was sentenced to life in prison without parole for attempted murder, aggravated rape and aggravated burglary, a crime he didn't commit.

After more than 3 decades in the Louisiana State Penitentiary, a maximum security prison with a violent reputation, the Innocence Project took up his case. Repeatedly, this legal non-profit organisation requested fingerprint comparisons and DNA testing that could prove Mr W's innocence but they were denied.

Eventually, in March 2019, the fingerprints found at the crime scene were submitted to the powerful fingerprint ID system. The fingerprints and the subsequent DNA tests finally proved that a man who'd committed other sexual assaults in the neighborhood was responsible for the crimes he was convicted of, according to the registry.

He was set free in **2019** after spending **almost 37 years** in the prison. "I knew I was innocent, I didn't commit the crime but being a poor black kid, I didn't have the ability to fight the state of Louisiana" said Mr AW after his release.

One study estimated that **up to 10,000 people** may be wrongfully convicted of serious crimes **in the US every year**. *(Refer:*

25

*"Qualitatively Estimating the Incidence of Wrongful Convictions",
Criminal Law Bulletin 48(2) [2012] 221—279).*

Even though he was wrongly convicted, and everybody that was involved in his case i.e. the police officers, the investigating officers, the prosecutors and the jury got it 100% wrong (not even 1% right), what is mind-blowing is that nobody would be held responsible for this error and nobody that involved in his case would even say sorry to him. In fact, some of them would have even been promoted or rewarded for a job well done.

A similar case was excellently portrayed in the film *Just Mercy (2019)*. It tells the true story of Mr W.M, an African-American man who was convicted of the 1986 murder of Ms R.M, a white woman. Mr W.M was totally innocent. He was not at the crime scene, did not know the victim and did not have any motive to kill her. **But he was framed by the authority and sentenced to death**, which was eventually dismissed.

<u>Case No. 6</u>
Mr BM,
The biggest Ponzi Scheme, USA.
The Financial System.

Mr BM, a well-respected financier, convinced thousands of investors to hand over their savings, falsely promising unusually high returns. To avoid having too many investors reclaim their "profits," Mr BM encouraged them to stay in the scheme and earn even more money. Even though the "investing strategies" used were very vague and secretive, which he claimed to protect their businesses, but all of his clients truly believed in him. *(Source: Google - The Biggest US Ponzi Scheme In History.)*

He was caught in December **2008** and charged with fraud, money laundering, perjury, and theft. He was sentenced to 150 years in prison for running the biggest fraudulent scheme in the U.S. history. The prosecutors estimated the fraud to be worth USD 64.8 billion based on the amounts in the accounts of Mr BM's 4,800 clients.

In 1999 before Mr. BM was caught, Mr HM, a financial analyst had informed The U.S. Securities and Exchange Commission (SEC) that he believed it was **legally and mathematically impossible** to achieve the gains Mr BM claimed to deliver. According to him, he only took **four minutes** to conclude that Mr BM's numbers did not add up, and **another minute** to suspect they were fraudulent.

Despite of his effort to show that Mr BM was lying, he was **ignored by various authorities for many years.** He even co-authored a book with the leader of his legal team titled *No One Would Listen,* which was published in **March, 2011**. The book details the frustrating efforts he and his legal team made over a ten-year period **to alert the government, the industry, and the press about Mr BM's fraud**.

I don't want to go into details about Mr BM's ponzi scheme. But what I want to highlight here is that the prospect of getting a lot of easy money changed the way a business was run even in the USA. A well-respected financier, who used to be the former non-executive chairman of the NASDAQ stock market manipulated the whole systems that he was very familiar with to gain as much profit as possible in the shortest time possible.

Case No. 7
'G2' War,
Mar to Dec, 2003,
No. of Deaths: 150,000 - 1,100,000.

One of the reasons that the G2 War started was the finding (?accusation) by an Intelligence Agency from one of the superpower country that the '**I**' government had a "massive stockpile" of biological weapons or famously known as a Weapon of Mass Destruction (WMD), even though they could not provide any concrete evidences.

17 years later, now we knew that it was just a lie. There were no Weapons of Mass Destruction found in the whole of the 'I' territory. But this simple false finding (?lie) caused hundreds of thousands of

innocent people to die, a country to be destroyed and millions of other people to suffer for the past 17 years until today.

Again, no one will be held responsible for this error or this lie, even though the Intelligence Agency and its superpower country got it 100% wrong, with millions of innocent people died or suffered from it.

THE AIMS OF THIS BOOK

The aims of this book are as follow:

1.   To explain about the conservative treatment for common medical problems and to try to avoid from doing unnecessary medical tests, procedures, treatment or surgeries.

2.   To explain that some of the common medical problems such as the headaches, migraines, dizzy spells, fainting attacks, neck-pain, back-pain, stomach pain, heart-burns, body-ache or tiredness especially in the young people are not because there are something wrong with their bodies or they have dangerous diseases inside their bodies. They could be perfectly normal.

3.   To explain about the Conservative Treatment vs. Active or Invasive Treatment. Most of the managements for simple medical complaints only involve simple conservative treatment or simple medication. They do not need to go for expensive investigations, invasive treatment or even operations.

4.   To explain especially to young people that they should not be worrying about having certain cancer or rare diseases. If they have never been admitted to the government hospitals, then the chances are that they are healthy. The chances of having rare cancer or diseases are very low which make screening for them not worthwhile.

CHAPTER 2

MEDICAL SCREENING II

'Doubt whom you will, but never yourself'.
- Christian Nestell Bovee

Medical or Health Screening

For those who want to know more about the Medical or Health Screening, I will give further information below. There are a few criteria that a good Medical Screening Programme should have:

1.	The test should be sensitive, specific, reproducible, validated and safe.
2.	The test should be acceptable to the patients.
3.	The distribution and cut-off points for the test should be known.
4.	The test is inexpensive.

Again, a Sensitive test or **Sensitivity** means that the test is able to correctly identify those with the disease, to give the **True Positive Rate**, and a Specific test or **Specificity** is the ability of those test to correctly identify those without the disease, to give the **True Negative Rate**, as explained in the first chapter.

Reproducible test means that the test is able to duplicate the same correct and consistent results over and over again by repeating the same test. Validated is a form of checking that something is officially true and acceptable. Safe test means that the screening test does not have any unacceptable side effects or complications.

The screening test should be simple, easy and pain-free so that most people would accept it. Some of the tests available even though they are very accurate such as the angiogram test to check for the Coronary Heart Disease, but it can be very dangerous and is not acceptable as a screening test.

Some of the screening tests unfortunately do not give 100% clear-cut results. It means that the distribution and cut-off points for the test are not that clear. These test results could be interpreted as suspicious, which means that the doctors are not sure whether they are normal or abnormal. These patients either need to repeat the tests, or do other tests to confirm these suspicious results, which require more and more further tests.

The screening test should also be cheap, so that the test can be done on a large number of people. For example a Chest X-Ray is a very good test to screen from Pulmonary Tuberculosis (PTB) infection. It is cheap, easy to take, painless, not dangerous and it will give the same result over and over again if it is repeated.

Unfortunately, in general there is no ideal screening method that has been discovered yet. In a study titled **'Screening tests: a review with examples'** by Drs L. Maxim, R. Niebo, and M. Utell (Ref: Inhal Toxicol. 2014 Nov; 26(13): 811–828.) gave the following remark: **Screening of asymptomatic populations is not always appropriate and could do more harm than good.**

MEDICAL EXAMINATION FOR MALAYSIAN PILOTS

I am one of the doctors that could do the medical examination for the Malaysian Pilots, either they are from the Malaysian Airlines, Air Asia, Malindo or a few other airlines. There are less than 40 doctors out of more than 70,000 doctors in the whole of Malaysia that have this aviation medical examiner certificate.

The medical examination reports and certificates that we sign are recognised by the International Civil Aviation Organization (ICAO), and our pilots can fly their aircrafts to the European countries as well as to the US.

We only do a few medical screening tests as advised by the Civil Aviation Authority of Malaysia (CAAM), who follows the standards set by the International Civil Aviation Organization (ICAO) every time we examine the pilots.

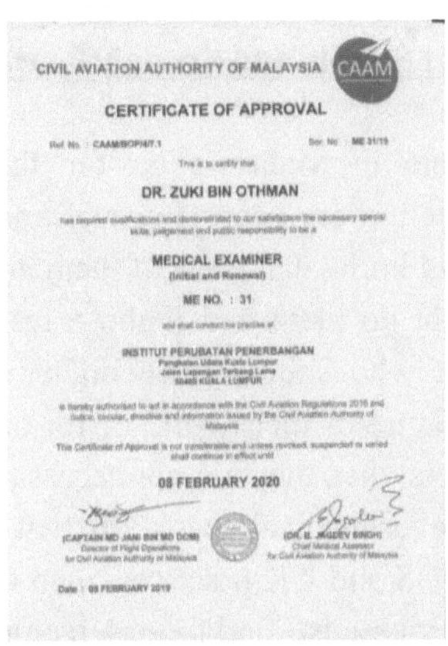

Picture-2: Medical Examiner Certificate for Civil Aviation Authority of Malaysia (CAAM).

Since it is very important that all the pilots have a good health standard, I also surprise to learn that not many tests are done for their yearly medical check-ups. The tests that we do for the pilots are as in Table-4 below:

SER	TESTS	BELOW 40 Y.O	40-60 Y.O	ABOVE 60 Y.O
1.	Medical Exam.	Every Year	Every Year	Every 6 Months
2.	Haemoglobin	Every Year	Every Year	Every 6 Months
3.	Urine Test	Every Year	Every Year	Every 6 Months
4.	Cholesterols	Every 5 years or if clinically indicated		
5.	Blood Sugar	Every 5 years or if clinically indicated		
6.	ECG	Every 5 years (<30) Every 2 years (<40)	Every Year	Every 6 Months
7.	Audiogram	Every 5 years	Every 2 years	Every 2 Years
8.	CXR	Every 5 years or if clinically indicated		

Table-4: The Medical Screening Tests for Malaysian Pilots.
(Source: Civil Aviation Authority of Malaysia (CAAM) - CEO Directives).

Despite of these lack of medical tests done for our pilots, I have never heard of any cases of the Malaysian Pilots collapsed, became incapacitated or had a heart attack during their flights.

a.   <u>**SM-3MM: Recommendations For The Medical Screening:
Keep It Simple and Straightforward-(KISS)**</u>

Many people in Malaysia go for their Medical or Health Screening Programme every year. However, most of these tests are not necessary. How do I know that most of them are unnecessary? Easy. If most doctors do not do them and if those tests are not done for our military personnel, who should have higher risks of having health issues due to the nature of their work, or for our Royal Malaysian Air Force (RMAF) pilots, then they are not necessary.

Since whatever medical check-ups that our military doctors do usually follow the US and UK practices, then the US and UK Military Medical Health Services also find these screening tests unnecessary.

Here are my recommendations for the **basic and simple tests** that you should do if you want to do a routine medical or health screening examination. These tests are almost the same with what our military doctors did for their military personnel when I was working there.

They might do more tests now to keep up with the easily available screening tests in Malaysia. These Screening Tests are for those who do not have any particular diseases or significant complaints.

If you already have any chronic diseases such as the Diabetes Mellitus (DM), Hypertension, Coronary Heart Diseases (CHD), Hepatitis B infections, Chronic Kidney problems or Cancer, then your regular doctors would advise what tests should be done periodically.

If you have other risks such as having multiple sexual partners then you should also check for the Sexually Transmitted Diseases (STDs), including for the Cervical Cancer in women.

From Tables-5 and 6 below, you can see that there are **not** many tests that you should do for your Health Screening Programme. For example, If you are a man who is less than 30 years old, then you only need to check for your blood pressure once a year. If it is normal, you just need to repeat it once every year, more if it is not normal. That is it.

Table-5: Recommended Tests for Men According To Age

AGE	BP	Urine FEME	CXR	ECG	Stress Test	U/S Abd	Sugar/ Lipids	Kidney /Liver	Others	Others
							BLOOD TESTS			
< 20	Medical Check Ups done at Schools / Pre-College Medical Check ups									
20+	Pre-College Medical Check-ups / Pre-Employment Medical Check Ups									
25+	1x /yr	1x/ 2-5yrs	1x/ 5-10 yrs	Nil	Nil	Nil	Nil	Nil	According to Risk factors	According to Risk factors
30+										
35+										
40+										
45+	2-3x /yr	1x/ yr	1x/ 5yrs	1x/ 5-10 yrs	May be once	1x/ 5-10 yrs	1x/ 5 yrs	1x/ 5 yrs		
50+										
55+										
60+				1x/ 2-5 yrs	1x/ 2-5 yrs	1x/ 5yrs	1x/ 2-3 yrs	1x/ 2-3 yrs		
65+										
70+										

Table-5: SM-3MM Recommended Tests for Men according To Age

Table-6: Recommended Tests for Women According To Age

AGE	BP	Urine (FEME)	CXR	ECG	Stress Test	Ultrasound Abdomen	Sugar/ Lipids	Kidneys /Liver	Others	Others
							BLOOD TESTS			
< 20	Enough with Medical Check Ups done at Schools / Pre-College Medical Check ups									
20+	Enough with Pre-College Medical Check-ups / Pre-Employment Medical Check Ups									
25+	1x/yr	1x/ 2-5yrs	1x/ 5-10 yrs	Nil	Nil	Nil	Nil	Nil	According to Risk factors	According to Risk factors
30+										
35+										
40+										
45+	2-3x /yr	1x/ yr	1x/ 5yrs	1x/ 5-10 yrs	May be once	1x/ 5-10 yrs	1x/ 5 yrs	1x/ 5 yrs		
50+										
55+										
60+				1x/ 5yrs	1x/ 5yrs	1x/ 5yrs	1x/ 2-3 yrs	1x/ 2-3 yrs		
65+										
70+										

Table-6: SM-3MM Recommended Tests for Women according To Age

I know that for some people these tests are too little. But that is what we did to our military personnel when I was working there. For example for young soldiers less than 40 years old, they only needed to check their health status once for every 4 years. We only checked their Physical Status, Blood Pressures, Urine tests and Chest X-rays. I have done less than the above recommendations for my own health screening tests.

For women, you need to be very careful with your suspicious results, for example from the Mammograms, Pap Smears, Ultrasounds of the abdomen or other tests. As I mentioned above regarding the Mammograms, for every 1,000 random Mammograms done in Malaysia we will get 98 suspicious results in normal women. These suspicious results in normal women would lead to more tests or procedures being done and sometimes they would even end up with unnecessary operations.

Since the number of the Cervical Cancer cases are less than the Breast Cancer, about 2,000 to 3,000 per year in Malaysia, and the results from the Pap Smears are more operator dependant, then there are more suspicious results in the Pap Smear tests compared to the Mammograms. These suspicious results would then lead to other unnecessary procedures or operations.

We would have the same problems with the ultra-sound tests. I have many patients who were perfectly normal with no signs and symptoms of any diseases, went for a routine ultrasound test but ended up with major surgical operations.

MEDICAL SECREENING FOR CHRONIC DISEASES

In my opinion, most people do unnecessary medical screening looking for the wrong medical problems. For example, if you are a young people that do not suffer from Hypertension or Diabetes, then you should not be doing blood tests, ultrasounds or other tests for the kidney problems, because the chance of you having the kidney problems is very low.

The Major causes of Kidney Failures in Malaysia are Diabetes (68%) and Hypertension (18%). There are at least 50 other diseases or factors that can cause the other 14% of Kidney Failures. Furthermore, we can detect for early kidney problems through a simple Urine test as advised above.

And if you are a young lady who is not menopausal, then you don't have to check for your cholesterol levels, or do bone scan for osteoporosis or check for the possible Coronary Heart Disease, because your oestrogen hormone will protect your heart and bones from the above diseases.

If you really want to do a medical screening, then you should just concentrate on the 4 main chronic diseases. These disease are:

1.   Diabetes Mellitus.

2.   Hypertension.

3.   Coronary Heart Disease (CHD).

4.   Cancer:

      a.   For men: Lung, Colorectal and Prostate Cancer.

      b.   For Women: Breast, Colorectal and Cervical Cancer.

SER	CHRONIC DISEASE	TESTS	AGE (years)				
			<20	<35	< 40	< 50	< 60
1.	DM	U.Sugar	-	1x/yr	1x/yr	1x/yr	1x/yr
		FBS	-	-	1x/yr	1x/yr	1x/yr
		HbA1c	-	-	-	1x/yr	1x/yr
2.	HPT	BP	-	1x/yr	1x/yr	1x/yr	2x/yr
3.	CHD	Lipids	-	-	1x/3yrs	1x/yr	1x/yr
		StressTest	-	-	-	If Ind.	If Ind.
		CT-Angio	-	-	-	If Ind.	If Ind.
4.	CANCER						
	a. Lung	CXR	-	-	-	1x/2yrs	1x/yr
	b. Breast	Br. Exam.	-	1x/yr	2x/yr	2x/yr	3x/yr
		Others	-	If Ind.	If Ind.	If Ind.	If Ind.
	c. Cervical	?PapSmear	-	-	If Ind.	If Ind.	If Ind.
		HPV-DNA	-	-	If Ind.	If Ind.	If Ind.
	d. Colon	FOB	-	-	If Ind.	If Ind.	If Ind.
		Sigmoid-oscopy	-	-	If Ind.	If Ind.	If Ind.
	e. Prostate	U/sound	-	-	-	-	1x/5yrs
		PSA	-	-	-	-	1x/2yrs

DM-Diabetes Mellitus, **U.Sugar**-Urine Sugar, **FBS**-Fasting Blood Sugar, **yr**-year, **HbA1c**-Glycated Haemoglobin (A1c), **HPT**-Hypertension, **BP**-Blood Pressure, **CHD**-Coronary Heart Disease, **CXR**-Chest X-Ray, **FOB**-Faecal Occult Blood, **PSA**-Prostate Specific Antigen

Table-7: Recommended Screening Tests For The Chronic Diseases For People With Average Risks For The Chronic Diseases. For People In The <u>High Risk Groups</u>, You Should Discuss With Your <u>Regular Doctors</u>.

1.   **<u>Diabetes Mellitus.</u>**

For Diabetes Mellitus, if you do not have a strong family history of Diabetes Mellitus, you can just check your Urine Glucose Test once every 2-3 years until you are 40 years old. After that you should check for your Urine Glucose Test together with the Fasting Blood Glucose (FBS) level preferably once a year.

If you have a strong family history of Diabetes Mellitus, then you should check for Urine Glucose Test once a year until you are 35 years old, then you should check for your Fasting Blood Glucose (FBS) and Urine Glucose Tests once a year.

There is another test called an HbA1c Test or Glycated Haemoglobin (A1c) Test, which is more accurate than the FBS test. You may do this test once a year after you are over 40 years old.

2.   **<u>Hypertension.</u>**

For Hypertension, it is very easy to check. You can just ask your regular doctor or your pharmacist to check your blood pressure once a year, more if they are not normal.

3.   **<u>Coronary Heart Disease (CHD).</u>**

For the Coronary Heart Disease (CHD), in general it is difficult to detect early. But if you are already suffering from Diabetes Mellitus or Hypertension, or both, or with a strong family history of Coronary Heart Disease then you are in the high risk group. Your regular doctor should monitor your heart more closely.

If you are not in this high risk group, for men you could just monitor your blood cholesterol level when you are 40 years old and above, and once you are menopausal for women, preferably once a year.

4.   **<u>Cancer.</u>**

    a.   **<u>Colorectal Cancer.</u>**

For Colorectal Cancer, again it is not easy to diagnose it early. But you should not be doing a colonoscopy test straight away to prevent from the **False Positive Finding**, where the doctor finds a lesion that looks like a cancer but it is not, unless you have a very strong family history of a colorectal cancer.

If you don't have a strong family history of a colorectal cancer, then you could start screening for the colorectal cancer if you have the following symptoms:

(1).   A persistent change in your bowel habits, including diarrhoea or constipation or a change in the consistency of your stool.

(2).   Rectal bleeding or blood in your stool.

(3).   Persistent abdominal discomfort, such as cramps, gas or pain.

(4).   A feeling that your bowel doesn't empty completely.

(5).   Weakness or fatigue.

(6).   Unexplained weight loss.

You could start with simple tests first, for eg. a Complete Blood Picture, a Fecal Occult Blood (FOB) stool test and a Sigmoidoscopy test. If they are positive or the symptoms and signs are persistent then you should do more tests, which include the Colonoscopy Test.

b.   <u>Breast Cancer.</u>

For Breast Cancer, you should do a regular breast examination for breast lumps. Any lump in the breast should be investigated, and preferably removed as early as possible.

As I have mentioned above, the mammogram test alone is not accurate. So do the CT-scan and ultrasound test. They can lead to False Positive Findings and lead to the unnecessary treatment.

If you have a very strong family history of Breast Cancer, then you should check for the BRCA1 and BRCA2 gene tests as well.

c.   **<u>Lung Cancer.</u>**

As for the lung cancer, there is no good screening test available to detect the lung cancer early. By the time we can see a lesion in the chest x-ray it is already too late. So it is better to prevent from getting the lung cancer than to screen for it.

Since 90% of the lung cancer cases are related to smoking, to stop smoking is the best way to prevent from getting a lung cancer.

d.   **<u>Prostate Cancer.</u>**

For Prostate Cancer, a Prostate-Specific Antigen (PSA) Blood Test is not accurate, as explained above. If you are really worried about having a Prostate Cancer then you can do a simple prostate ultra-sound test for an enlarged prostate.

Since they are not that common in the young people and the incidence rate is not that high, you may check for the prostate cancer if you have the following symptoms:

(1).   Frequent urination (not due to Diabetes).

(2).   Weak or interrupted urine flow or the need to strain to empty the bladder.

(3).   The urge to urinate frequently at night.

(4).   Blood in the urine.

(5).   New onset of Erectile Dysfunction (ED).

(6).   Discomfort or pain when sitting, caused by an enlarged prostate.

e.   **<u>Cervical Cancer.</u>**

For Cervical Cancer, again, a pap smear alone is not accurate, as I have explained above. If you are not in the high risk group of having the Cervical Cancer for e.g. you do not have multiple sexual partners and family history of Cervical Cancer, then you can start taking the tests after having the following signs and symptoms:

(1).   Blood spots or light bleeding between or following periods.

(2).   Menstrual bleeding that is longer and heavier than usual.

(3).   Bleeding after intercourse, douching, or a pelvic examination.

(4).   Increased vaginal discharge.

(5).   Pain during sexual intercourse.

(6).   Bleeding after menopause.

(7).   Unexplained, persistent pelvic and/or back pain.

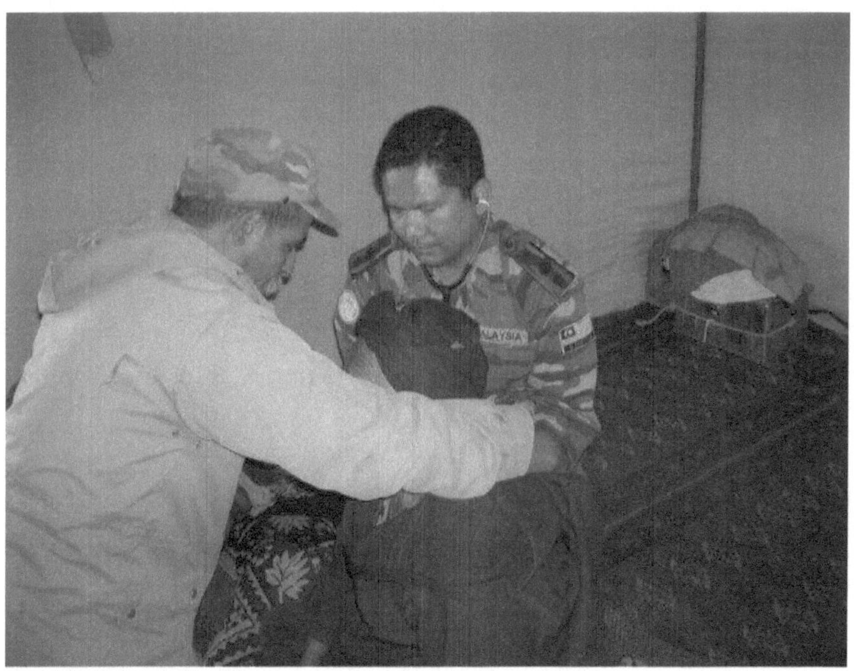

Picture-3: Giving Free Medical Treatment to Local People.

CHAPTER 3

MAKING SENSE OF THE MEDICAL TREATMENT

'The art of medicine consists in amusing the patient while nature cures the disease'.

- *Voltaire*

I believe that for most people, the treatment that they are getting when they get sick, either at the government hospitals or at the private hospitals sometimes are very confusing and puzzling. Most of the time they are not sure whether they are getting too much or too little of the treatment or the investigations from either of these hospitals.

For example, say that they are having high fevers for one or two weeks, together with other common complaints such as the coughs, a runny nose, a sore throat, headaches, body pain or rashes. At the government hospitals or clinics, they usually have to wait for a few hours as the clinics are usually very busy.

Most of the time the doctors at the government clinics tend not to do any tests, instead they would immediately treat the complaints. Usually they will be diagnosed with a simple diagnosis such as a Common Cold, a Flu or a Viral Fever, or with an Acute Upper Respiratory Tract Infection (URTI).

Sometimes, the diagnosis can be a little bit more specific, like a Bronchitis in an adult or a Bronchiolitis in a children. However, these diagnoses are still general diagnoses, which mean the same thing i.e. **common viral respiratory tract infections**. They do not pinpoint to any specific causes or organisms.

They are then given with simple medication, usually without any antibiotics. They will be advised to go back home and rest, and to come back to the clinic or hospital if and when necessary. Sometimes they are not even given any medical certificates (MCs) or sick-leaves at all. Instead, they are asked to go back to work.

That's it. Yes, that is all the treatment that they are getting from the government clinics. All of that after having the above symptoms for more than a week, and after waiting for a few hours for the treatment.

In contrast, with less of these symptoms and if they go to the private medical facilities, suddenly they would have many tests done. At the private clinics or hospitals, they cannot be seen to treat the patients like the way they are being treated at the government clinics. Otherwise why bother going to the private medical centers. Again, Many people believe that doing more tests or seeing more specialists are better. They would have their blood and urine tests done. Sometimes these tests would include the x-rays, ultra-sounds or even the MRIs and CT-scans.

They would then be immediately diagnosed with a scary disease or an infection. For example with an Influenza A or H1N1 infection, or an Influenza B infection, or with difficult to pronounce viruses like a Respiratory Syncytial Virus (RSV) or an Adenovirus infection, and sometimes are advised to be admitted to the hospitals for immediate treatment.

I would like to stress here from the beginning that we have one of the best private health care services in the world. Yes, it is true and we should be proud of it. Malaysia has been awarded **"Destination of the Year"** for health care travel for 5 years in a row from **2015 to 2019** by the **International Medical Travel Journal (IMTJ).**
(Refer: https://awards.imtj.com/results/)

International Living, another international publication for subscribers detailing the best places in the world to live, retire, travel, and invest, has ranked Malaysia as No. 1 in the Best Health-care in the World category of the 2019 International Living Annual Global Retirement Index. *(Source: The Star newspaper dated 07 Feb 2019)*

For 2019, here is what Cision PRWeb has to say about Malaysia:

1.   Scoring 95 out of 100, Malaysia takes the top spot in the health care category of the International Living 2019 Annual Global Retirement Index. The health care in the Southeast Asian gem is simply world class with up-to-date and sophisticated infrastructure.

2.   There are 13 **Joint Commission International** (**JCI**)- accredited hospitals in the country and almost every doctor is fluent in English. In fact, most Malaysian doctors were trained in the UK, U.S., or Australia so communication is flawless. It's not surprising Malaysia a popular tourism destination.

3.   Here, you don't need an appointment to see a specialist, and you don't need a referral from a general practitioner either. It's as simple as registering at a hospital and waiting in line to see your specialist of choice.

4.   Prescriptions in Malaysia cost a fraction of the U.S. prices. But it's not just the cost that's attractive- it's the service. The pharmacists, like the rest of Malaysia's medical staff, are well trained and informed. Malaysians are friendly people, but it's the genuine interest that they take which impresses.

5.   "Recently, I decided on a whim to have a medical wellness exam," says Mr K.H, IL Malaysia Correspondent. "I'd never had one done before and as I had a free morning I decided just to pop in to the LWE Hospital," says Mr K.H, who lives on the island of Penang.

6.   "I was already registered and found myself sitting outside a doctor's office not five minutes after arriving. Within an hour, I had been examined by a doctor, had an ECG and blood and urine tests done…and I was on my way home.

7.   "The total cost of the visit was just USD44 (RM183). The doctor who had examined me called me later that afternoon with the results. It's this level of service that makes medical care in Malaysia an attractive option. It's all so easy."

We also have excellent private clinics or General Practioners (GPs), pharmacies and private laboratory services in Malaysia. You can go and see any one of the GPs at anytime you like, sometimes they are even available 24 hours a day, and do many of the blood and urine tests or x-rays at the same time. The results of the x-rays would be available immediately, and the results of the blood and urine tests would be available within 1 to 3 days.

If you go to the United Kingdom (UK), it will take from a few days to a few weeks just to make an appointment to see their General Practitioners. Even with the appointments, you still need to wait, sometimes for hours to see your doctor. And you would **NOT** be able to do most of the tests that you would like to do if there are no indications for those tests.

The problem with the Malaysian system is that if you start abusing the system. Then there will be many problems and complications that would arise from these abuses, which I will discuss more in this book. These problems are not only peculiar to the health systems. They can also happen to other systems as well, for e.g. the banking systems.

In the banking systems all over the world, they have very strict procedures before they could approve any loans to the borrower. But during the **sub-prime mortgage crisis in the US in 2007** as an example, they abused one simple rule, by giving housing loans to the people that have low credit ratings i.e. people that could not afford to pay back the loans. By abusing this simple, basic rule, the sub-prime mortgage crisis caused several major US financial institutions to collapse in September 2008, and triggered the onset of a **severe global recession**.

Another example of the different treatment between the government and private medical services is a back pain. It is another common complaint at the General Practitioner's (GP) clinic. Most of the time at the government clinics or hospitals you will be given pain-killers, massage oils or creams and that is it. You will not be given any more appointments except to come again if necessary. Rarely would they send you for a physiotherapy treatment as their physiotherapy units are usually packed with more severe cases.

In comparison, if you go to the private sectors, again they would do more that what the government hospitals do. Immediately they would do back or lumbar-sacral x-rays, or neck x-rays if the pain is higher up. Most of the time they would also do the MRI scans and again come up with a scary and alarming diagnosis, such as a Slipped Disc.

With these Slipped Discs, some people think that they might lead to other severe complications, such as leading to paralysis of their limbs. The thoughts that they would need further treatment to repair their slipped discs and prevent them from having paralysis of their limbs would lead to other medical procedures to treat the slipped discs such as the steroid injections or operations.

I am very surprised to find out that they are so many people that have gone for the back or neck operations and the steroid injections for their slipped discs. (I will discuss more about the slipped discs in Chapter 6 of this book.)

If I were not a doctor, I would have done the same thing. I have many similar complaints like many normal Malaysians do. I think I would have had an abdominal x-ray, ultrasound, endoscopy and colonoscopy done for my gastritis and constipation, a chest x-ray, an MRI or a CT scan of the chest or even a bronchoscopy done for my chronic cough, back x-rays and MRIs for my back pain and many more.

Since I am a doctor, I do not need to do any of the above tests. My symptoms are not bad enough to require me to go for all those investigations. Even if I were to have all those tests done, we already knew that either the results were normal or they would have been insignificant to require for more aggressive treatment. Therefore, the above investigations are not necessary. I will just take simple medication to treat all of my problems.

<u>**Case No. 8**</u>

Dr A,

A Professor and Consultant Physician,

UK.

You would probably be surprised if I say that most doctors are the same as or even more conservative than I am. One of my friends,

Dr A decided to stay and started working in Ireland and UK after he completed his medical degree in 1995. When he was young, he was very active physically playing basketball, volleyball, badminton and many other sports.

He had put on a lot of weight especially during his specialist training as most of his time were spent at the hospitals. When he eventually became a consultant at one of the leading university hospitals in England he decided to start running. Unfortunately, every time he tried to run he would complain of severe pain in both of his knees.

He went to see his orthopaedic friend. After the examinations and MRI scans, his friend concluded that he had severe ligament tears in both of his knee joints. Being an experienced orthopaedic surgeon, his friend reassured him that he could repair the tears. Moreover, the operation would be free as Dr A was working with the UK National Health Service (NHS).

However, since his problem was not a life-threatening problem, like many other doctors, Dr A refused the operation. He did not want his body to be subjected to any strong drugs or major operations. He started running anyway after putting plenty of straps at his knee joints and wearing good knee supports.

It was very difficult and very painful in the beginning. However, he was very persistent with his running activities. When I met him one day he had been running every day for almost 2 years. He managed to reduce his weight by 50%. Now he can run in a full marathon including the London Marathon and Boston Marathon, even with severe ligament tears in both of his knees.

<u>Case No. 9</u>

Dr B,

A Consultant O&G,

Malaysia.

Some other doctors can be more extreme than that. One day Dr B, an Obstetric and Gynaecologist (O&G) specialist who was one of my wife's friends had a big swelling in one of her breasts, which we call an abscess. Since she also had a fever, and with that big abscess, she was advised to go for an Incision and Drainage (I & D) operation under a general anaesthesia at the hospital.

Like most doctors, the thought of going for a procedure or an operation that involve several strong drugs injected into her body and to put her life under somebody else hands were too much for her. She decided to do it herself. She took the alcohol swabs, a scalpel with a surgical blade, gauzes, cotton balls and a few other things back home. She cut open her abscess and cleaned it herself.

<u>Treatment For Private Patients</u>

I am not saying that this is the correct way of treating your medical problems. **If fact, this is the wrong way**. However, most doctors will not simply go for any procedures or operations unless they are very necessary. Unfortunately, I have many patients that are very happy and very eager to go and see the specialists or to be admitted to the hospitals even for minor medical problems. Sometimes they even insist on getting a few letters to go and see a few different specialists.

Once I had a 40-something lady who requested three different referral letters to see three different specialists. She wanted to see an orthopaedic surgeon for her back pain, a gynaecologist for her woman's health check-up and another specialist, which I did not remember what it was for. In that one day she was referred to more specialists than my grandfather, my father and I had ever seen in our entire lives (228 years combined).

Since many of the medical tests are not accurate, in some of these referred cases, they would end up with other procedures that are more invasive, or even would end up with surgeries where some of them are unnecessary. Some of these major surgeries are very difficult, complicated and complex.

Once I had a middle-aged man who went for a back operation for his back pain in Kuala Lumpur, but needed to go for two other back operations to correct the complications from the first operation. Even after these three operations, his backache was still there.

Another young woman went for two operations to remove her ovarian cysts. Unfortunately, she continued to have abdominal pain whenever she had her menstrual period. She had another ultra-sound test done, and found to have a new cyst. She believed that her period pain would never be resolved unless the doctors keep removing the cysts surgically. One young man ended up with an endoscopy, a colonoscopy and an appendicectomy done for his abdominal pain.

In the government hospitals, all these cases would have been treated with simple pain-killers or with other conservative treatment **first**. However, most of these patients believed that pain-killers would never cure their problems unless they remove the causes, which are **not the best practice in medicine.**

Some of the patients even have their own consultants, for eg. their own gynaecologist, or their own surgeons. In contrast, my grandmother who died in her 70s and my mother who is more than 70 years old now have never seen any gynaecologists their entire lives.

My wife, a Professor at one of the Public Medical School and is over 50 years old, also refuses to see any gynaecologists, even though she has many friends and colleagues who work as gynaecologists. Again, I have to stress here that she does not want to see the gynaecologists not because she does not trust them. She does not want to see them because she does not have enough signs and symptoms that justify her for a gynaecological examination.

Even in the UK, they will not allocate a personal gynaecologist to their patients. What they do is to refer you to a gynaecology team where a group of doctors in that team will see you. What they practice in the UK is for you to have your own **General Practitioner (GP).**

By having your own GP, you will be seeing the same doctor every time you need to see a doctor. They hope by doing that, your regular GP will be more likely to pick up any significant medical problems that you might have, **and refer you to the specialists only if the findings are significant, or relevant.**

So, regarding the young patients that came to my clinics complaining of frequent headaches, migraines, dizzy spells, fainting attacks, neck pain, back pain, stomach pain, heartburns, body-ache or tiredness, usually I would try to stop them from continuing their complaints. I would try to tell them that most probably all the normal results that they were getting were right. Which meant that there were nothing wrong with them. Most probably all these symptoms were due to the psychological stress, or work stress or personal problems.

Don't get me wrong. I am not against modern medical treatment. In fact, **I only believe in the modern medicine**. Therefore, I do not believe in any of the complementary medicine. I do not believe in the homeopathy, traditional medicine, naturopathy and Ayurveda, mind and body practices like acupuncture and massage therapy, the natural health products like herbs, dietary supplements or probiotics. How could I believe in these complementary medicine since they go against basic science?

One of the aims of this book is to give my readers a different view of the medical treatment for some of their medical problems. This is not a new form of the medical treatment. This is what the government hospitals in Malaysia are practising and what the doctors in the UK are practising.

In the medical world, we call this practice as *The Best Practice in Medicine*. The private clinics and hospitals in Malaysia also practice the same *Best Practice in Medicine,* but we need to have 2 extra things in mind, to please the patients and to gain profits.

<u>BEST PRACTICE</u>

So, what is a Best Practice in Medicine? This is one of the explanations that I could find on the internet. ***A best practice in Medicine is a method or technique that has been generally accepted as superior to any alternatives, because it produces results that are superior to those achieved by other means or because it has become a standard way of doing things that comply with legal or ethical requirements.***

Unfortunately, most doctors do not talk or explain enough about this to the common people, or they are not writing enough about it. Well, that is what the Best Practice means. To put it simply, it means that the treatment given is **the best standard treatment given to a patient, which complies with legal or ethical requirements.**

We cannot compare human beings or human bodies to machines. In machines, yes, for most of the problems they are better if we could rectify the problems earlier. It is very different with our bodies. Therefore, we cannot use our usual logic to request for investigations, procedures or treatment for our common medical problems.

Definitely we cannot use *google* to find out what is wrong with our bodies and what tests or procedures need to be done. We need to use the Best Practice Guidelines. In most of the simple or moderately severe medical problems, ***our bodies have the ability to heal ourselves***. In these cases, we should just use simple treatment, and let our bodies heal themselves.

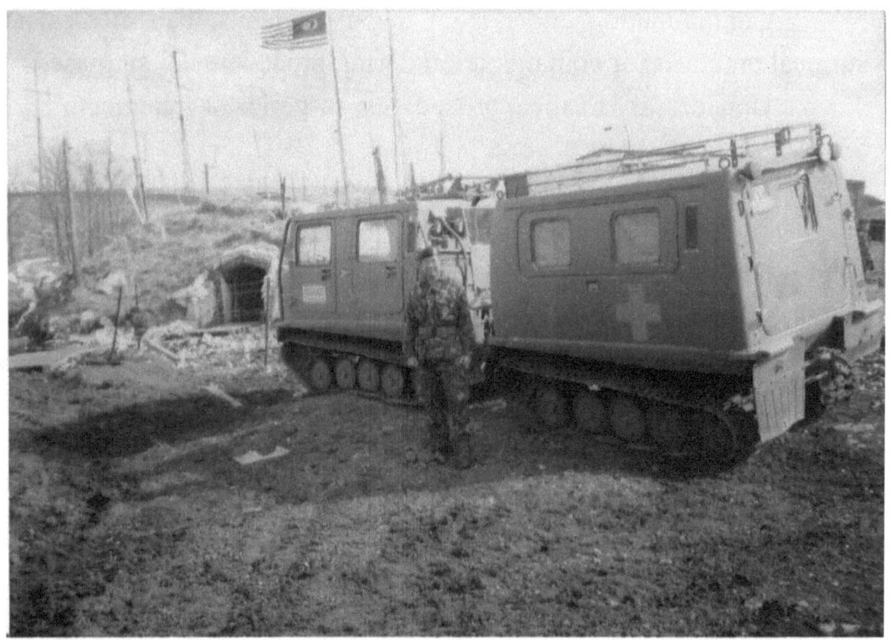

Picture-4: ..with An Ambulance, Livno, Bosnia-Herzegovina.

CHAPTER 4

IATROGENIC PROBLEMS

'Isn't it a bit unnerving that doctors call what they do "practice"?'
-        *George Carlin*

Iatrogenic Problems are medical problems due to the side effects of the medication, activities of the doctors, or due to the complications from the procedures and surgeries. It came from a Greek word Iatrogenesis, which means "brought forth by the healer".

So in general, the possible iatrogenic problems include:

1.   Side effects from the medication or from multiple drug interactions.

2.   Complications from the medical procedures, surgeries or treatment.

3.   Contamination either from the instruments, bad medical and surgical practices, or contamination during procedures or surgeries.

4.   Unnecessary medical procedures, surgeries or treatment.

5.   Medical Errors.

6.   Medical Negligence.

Iatrogenic problems are unavoidable. No hospitals in the world could guarantee that there will not be any iatrogenic problems or medical errors at their hospitals. What they can do is to reduce these iatrogenic problems. The true extent of the cost of this problem to the health system or to human mortality and morbidity is difficult to measure.

The reason is that the health personnel would not just want to admit that the patients are getting worse due to the faults that occur at their hospitals or due to their faults. If they don't admit, then there won't be any records of these errors or problems. It is the same with other professions.

A Prime Minister or a President would not want to admit that the country's economy is getting worse because of him. He would blame other things first like the oil price, the Chinese government, the weather phenomenon like the El-Nino or La-Nina, the previous governments or on something else.

It does not mean that we should avoid the modern treatment because of these iatrogenic problems. We should not stop driving a car or riding a motorcycle because every year in Malaysia about 15,000 people die or suffer serious injuries due to the Road Traffic Accidents (RTAs). Definitely we should not start riding horses or camels to reduce these deaths or serious injuries.

If we stop practising modern treatment, more people would die or become worse from the illnesses or from other form of treatment. What we need to do is either to avoid the possible causes of the iatrogenic problems or try to reduce them.

A study done in the US by Drs Martin Makary and Michael Daniel and published by the **British Medical Journal** (BMJ) in **2016** using a complex mathematical model or analysis put medical error as the third leading cause of deaths in the US in 2013, as shown in Table-7 below. *(Source: Refer BMJ 2016;353:i2139).*

SER	CAUSES	NO. OF DEATHS (Total: 2,596,993)	%
1.	Heart Disease	611,105	23.5
2.	Cancer	585,000	22.5
3.	*Medical Error*	*251,000*	*9.7%*
4.	Chronic Obstructive Pulmonary Disease (COPD)	149,000	5.7
5.	Stroke	128,978	5.0

Table-7: Leading Causes of Death in the US in 2013.

The fact that this article was published in the prestigious **British Medical Journal (BMJ)** meant that it was a highly credible research project. To estimate the number of deaths due to the iatrogenic causes at no. 3 was really significant. At 251,000 deaths, it represented about 9.67% of all deaths in the US in 2013.

If we could have deaths due to the iatrogenic causes, then we could also have serious, moderate and mild illnesses due to them. Some of these iatrogenic problems could be prevented if we could reduce the numbers of the unnecessary medical screening, medical procedures or the unnecessary operations.

That is why most doctors like Dr A and Dr B in Cases No. 8 and 9 above were very conservative with what type of treatment that they were getting with the type of medical problems that they had. Many of the major surgeries such as the heart operations, spine operations and brain surgeries are very difficult, complex and complicated to perform. They could also give rise to many bad complications as what happen to Mr C below.

<u>Case No. 10</u>
Mr C,
A 35-year-old Malaysian Business Consultant.

Mr C went to one of the private hospitals in Kuala Lumpur in July 2015, complaining of a back pain. The doctor that examined him recommended that he be admitted immediately for an urgent Magnetic Resonance Imaging (MRI)-test. After the MRI result was out, the doctor told him that he had suffered from a slipped disc in his thoracic region, which require a surgical treatment. *(Source: Google- A Malaysian Business Consultant back surgery left him a quadriplegic).*

However, the surgery didn't go as planned. The spine surgeon removed (?reason) 14 cm of his rib, severing his thoracic nerve and caused a permanent nerve damage. This initial problem in the operation made the doctor to abort the spine operation. He was discharged in a wheelchair, unable to walk.

He was later readmitted to the same hospital for a spinal fusion operation. Unfortunately the operation was also unsuccesful and left him a quadriplegic (paralysis of all four limbs), permanent nerve damage and life-changing disabilities.

Now he is bound to a wheelchair, requires regular medical treatment with medication to control muscle spasms, and daily rehabilitation sessions which are often interrupted by periods of illness, infection or depression.

Complications From A Simple Case

The treatment that you are getting from the hospitals, either at the government or private hospitals are stronger, more invasive and have higher risks of complications from what you are getting from the GP's clinics. That is why a government hospital will not admit any patient unless it is very necessary. Sometimes, even a simple case that is admitted to the hospital will go terribly wrong, as in the case below.

Case No. 11
Girl A,
An 11 year-old girl.

This case happened a few years ago. One day I had to cover for my partner at one of our clinics. That morning, my staff told me that the father of one of the patients that came to the clinic a few days earlier wanted to see the doctor. When I checked her record, she came a few days earlier complaining of the Common Cold symptoms i.e. a fever, coughs, a runny nose and a sore throat. Her body temperature was normal. He wanted to get my opinion on what went wrong in the treatment of his daughter which caused his daughter's death.

My young partner had given her all the possible medication that could be given to her i.e. Paracetamol tablets for the fever, a cough syrup for the cough, anti-histamine tablets for the runny nose, lozenges for the sore throat and even the antibiotics. Usually I did not agree with any doctors who just simply give the antibiotics. However, at that moment I was glad that she did. Which meant that the father could not fault us with any accusations such as being late in giving the antibiotics.

The father was working as a medical insurance agent. Even without a referral letter, he knew how to get his kids admitted to the hospitals. It was his common practice to get his kids admitted to the private hospitals if the complaints were not resolved after a few days. That day, a different paediatrician from his normal paediatric specialist that treats his kids treated his daughter. This specialist told him that his daughter needed to be admitted to the ICU, but unfortunately she died there.

I have many parents that insist their children to be admitted to the hospitals if they are not getting well after a few days of having the Common Cold symptoms. **This is wrong. The hospital is the last place to go for a Common Cold infection**. If the body temperature is normal or not persistently high, never send your children to the hospital. Give them plenty of fluid and let them rest at home.

I don't want to speculate about this case but we can learn a few things here:

1. The government hospital will never admit any patients that suffer from the Common Cold infections with a normal temperature. Because of this, the patient should had never ended up in the ICU.

2. The treatment at the private hospital is different compared to the treatment given at the government hospital. They are very swift, fast and give stronger treatment. These characteristics are good in real emergencies, but they could increase the complications or iatrogenic problems arising from these treatment. This girl should have been alive had she not been admitted to the hospital.

3. She died due to the complications from either the procedures or the treatment at the ICU, not from the Common Cold, because the common cold infections never cause any deaths in Malaysia (Chapter 8).

Treatment cure the problems - but give rise to other problems.

Sometimes, the treatment given for a particular medical problem would solve the problem, but it would give rise to other complications which are more severe and more debilitating than the problem that the treatment solved.

<u>Case No. 12</u>
Miss F,
A Medical Student.

One of my wife' students suffered from severe sweaty hands, which in a medical term it is called a hyperhidrosis. As a medical student, she needs to examine the patients, but with severe sweaty hands it would make the patients very uncomfortable. Therefore she went to see a Spine Surgeon for a further treatment.

The Spine Surgeon offered to do a surgery to cure the problem. The surgery which was done in **Jan 2018** was successful, and it cured her sweaty hands. Unfortunately she developed a severe and constant pain at the site of the operation at her back and severe sweating over her chest and back. Even though the sweaty chest and back were very uncomfortable, but the chronic pain that gave the most problems to her. The pain was so severe that she could not sleep, unless she was really tired and sleepy. Sometimes she could not sleep for a few days.

She was given with many different types of **strong pain-killers** and **sleeping tablets**, but they did not reduce her pain or make her fall to sleep. One day while she was driving and after not sleeping for a few days, **she crashed her car into a tree**. Luckily the injuries were not substantial. She also developed a depression and other personality disorders due to the constant chronic back pain, inability to sleep and the sweaty body. She was even referred to a few different psychiatrists and psychologists for her depression and personality disorders.

Eventually she was referred to a '*MENANG*' Pain Management Programme in March, 2019 after more than 1 year of suffering the above complications. (*MENANG* in the Malaysian national language means "win" and the name comes from the "*Program MENANGani Kesakitan*" which is translated into the **"Pain management Program"**). *Menang* is a multidisciplinary **Cognitive Behavioral Therapy** (CBT) intervention that can be effective for pain management therapy without giving any medicine to the patients.

CBT is a psychotherapy that combines cognitive therapy with behavior therapy by identifying faulty or maladaptive patterns of thinking, emotional response, or behavior and substituting them with desirable patterns of thinking, emotional response, or behavior.

In other words they were taught to control their pain by using their minds. **Yes, it is correct, they were taught to control their chronic pain by using their minds.** *(Refer: Self-management of chronic pain in Malaysian patients: effectiveness trial with 1-year follow-up. Website: https://www.ncbi.nlm.nih.gov/pmc/articles/PMC3291846/)*

Not everybody would be successful with this form of treatment. Fortunately she was one of those that were lucky to have their problems solved. Now she is able to control her pain and to sleep at night without taking any pain-killers or sleeping tablets. But she is still left with the sweaty chest and back, which she will need to endure for the rest of her life.

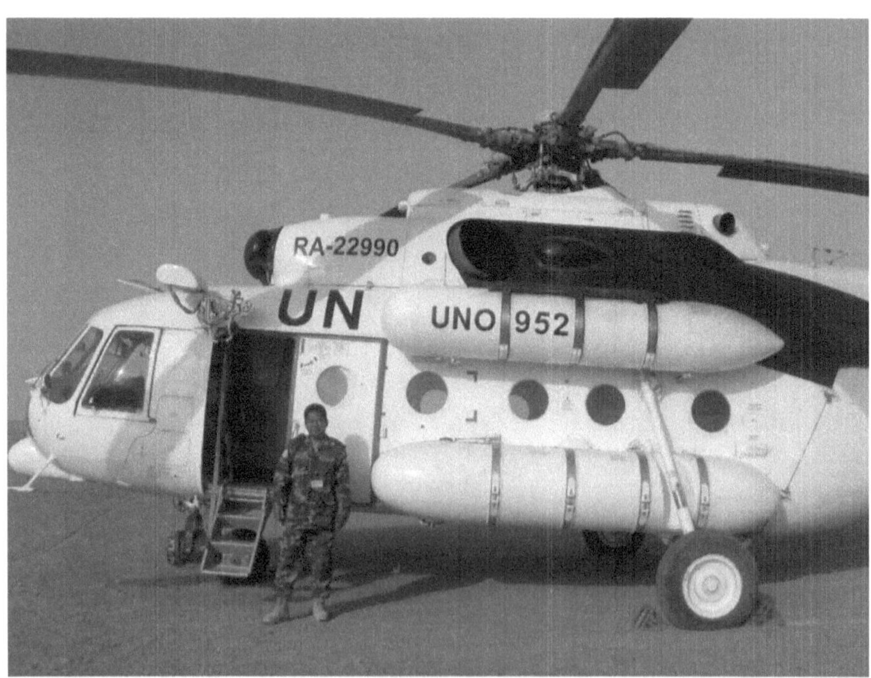

Picture-5: Our Usual Mode of Transport, which was also used as an Ambulance in Western Sahara.

CHAPTER 5

THE CHOOSING WISELY PROJECT

'As to diseases, make a habit of two things - to help, or at least, to do no harm.'

-        *Hippocrates*

The Choosing Wisely project was first launched in **2012** in the United States of America (USA) by the foundation of the American Board of Internal Medicine (ABIM). Initially it recruited nine medical specialty societies representing more than 376,000 doctors, which include the Family Physicians, the Cardiologists, the Radiologists, the Gastro-enterologists, the Oncologists, the Kidney specialists, the Specialists in Allergy, Asthma and Immunology and the Nuclear Cardiologist. *(Source-* Go to: *http://www.choosingwisely.org/our-mission).*

The reason they started this project was to promote conversations between doctors and patients by helping patients choose care that was:

1.   supported by evidence.
2.   not duplicate of other tests or procedures already received.
3.   free from harm.
4.   they were truly necessary.

Their aim was to reduce or eliminate unnecessary and sometimes harmful tests, procedures or treatment. Every year the US spends more than USD 3 trillion on health care, with spending in 2018 at USD 3.5 trillion and projected to be at USD 3.6 trillion in 2019. They estimated that waste in the total health care expenditure is between USD 760 billion to USD 935 billion annually, or about 25% of the total medical spending. These wastage are due to multiple factors, such as health insurance and medical uncertainties that encourage the production of inefficient and low-value services.

Now they have more than 80 medical specialty societies involved in this project with more than 1 million doctors. This means that majority of the doctors in the US support the Choosing Wisely Project. They also have a smart phone app, which can be downloaded for free into your handphone. So far, they have come up with more than 550 recommendations either to the doctors or to the patients. You can go to their websites and download their recommendations or install their apps in your smart phone.
(Go to: *http://www.choosingwisely.org/).*

By 2020, the choosing wisely projects or campaigns have spread to other countries such as the United Kingdom (UK), France, Germany, Norway, Australia, New Zealand, Ireland, Austria, Italy, Japan, Brazil and India. Their recommendations are very similar to my recommendations in this book.

In choosing wisely campaigns, they advocate their patients to ask five questions to their health care providers. For them *some tests, treatment and procedures provide little benefit. And in some cases, they may even cause harm.* Use the five questions to make sure you end up with the right amount of care - not too much and not too little.

These five questions are:

1.   **Do I really need this test, treatment or procedure?** Tests may help you and your doctor or other health care providers determine the problems. Treatment, such as medicine and procedures may help to treat them. However some of these tests, treatment or procedures are sometimes unnecessary.

2.   **What are the risks?** Will there be side effects to the tests or treatment? What are the chances of getting results that aren't accurate? Could that lead to more testing, additional treatment or other procedures?

3.   **Are there simpler, safer options?** Are there alternative options to treatment that could work. Lifestyle changes such as eating healthier foods or exercising more, can be safer and effective option.

4.   **What happens if I don't do anything?** Ask if your condition might get worse- or better - if you don't have the test, treatment or procedure done right away.

5.   **What are the costs?** Costs can be financial, emotional or a cost of your time. Where there is a cost to the community, is the cost reasonable or is there a cheaper alternative?

Examples of the recommendations given to the doctors and to the patients in the choosing wisely project are as follow:

1.   **Back Pain.**

   a.   **To Doctors.**

   (1).   Don't recommend imaging (i.e. Back X-rays, MRIs or CT-scans) of the spine within the first 6 weeks of an acute episode of low back pain in the absence of red flags (such as injuries from a Road Traffic Accident or a fall from a high building, a cancer with bony metastases or a bladder or a bowel dysfunction). -*North American Spine Society.*

   (2).   Avoid Imaging Studies (i.e. X-rays, MRIs or CT-scans) for Acute Low Back Pain without specific indications. -*American Society of Anesthesiologists - Pain Medicine.*

   b.   **To Patients.**

   (1).   You probably don't need an X-ray, MRI or CT-Scan for a back pain. Here's why:

   (a).   The tests will not help you feel better faster.

   (b).   Imaging tests have risks.

   (c).   Imaging tests are expensive.

   (d).   **Doing Imaging tests may lead to other unnecessary tests, procedures or even surgeries.**

   (2).   Usually, X-rays aren't needed for low back pain. X-rays should only be ordered if the patient has relevant symptoms. For example, a patient has a:

   (a).   Fever.

   (b).   History of injury.

   (c).   Significant loss of ability.

(d).   Bone condition.

2. **<u>Headache/ Concussion.</u>**
   a. **<u>To Doctors.</u>**
      (1).   Don't do imaging (i.e. X-rays, MRIs or CT-scans) for uncomplicated headache. *-American Society of Radiology.*
      (2).   Avoid CT-scan of the head in asymptomatic adult patients in the emergency department with syncope, insignificant trauma and a normal neurological evaluation. *- American College of Emergency Physicians.*
   b. **<u>To Patients.</u>**
      (1).   Imaging tests rarely help. Doctors see many patients with headache. And most of them have migraines or headaches caused by tension. Both kinds of headaches can be very painful. But a CT scan or an MRI rarely shows why the headache occurs. And they do not help you ease the pain.
      (2).   Brain scans are usually not helpful for a concussion.
      (3).   A CT scan takes pictures to create images of the brain. The scan can show if there's a fracture or bleeding. An MRI creates clear images of the brain tissue. But these scans cannot show if you have a concussion. A concussion affects how your brain works, and most people recover within a few weeks.

3. **<u>Colds, Flu, and Other Respiratory Illnesses.</u>**
   a. **<u>To Doctors.</u>**
      (1).   Avoid prescribing antibiotics for upper respiratory infections. *- American Society of Infectious Disease.*
      (2).   Antibiotics should not be used for viral respiratory illnesses **(sinusitis, pharyngitis, bronchitis or bronchiolitis)**. *-American Academy of Pediatric.*

b.   <u>**To Patients.**</u>

(1).   If you have a sore throat, cough, or sinus pain, you might expect to take antibiotics. After all, you feel bad, and you want to get better fast. But antibiotics don't help most respiratory infections, and they can even be harmful.

(2).   Overuse of antibiotics is a serious problem. Wide use of antibiotics breeds 'superbugs'. These are bacteria that become resistant to antibiotics. They can cause drug-resistant infections, even disability or death. The resistant bacteria -'the superbugs'- can also spread to family members and others.

4.   <u>**Cancer Screening.**</u>

a.   <u>**To Doctors.**</u>

(1).   Don't routinely use breast MRI for breast cancer screening in average risk women.

(2).   Don't recommend screening for breast, colorectal or Prostate Cancer if life expectancy is estimated to be less than 10 years.-*AMDA- The Society for Post-Acute and Long Term Care Medicine.*

(3).   Do not repeat colorectal cancer screening (by any methods) for 10 years after a high-quality colonoscopy that does not detect cancer.

b.   <u>**To Patients.**</u>

(1).   The Prostate-Specific Antigen (PSA) blood test can do more harm than good. Men under 50 or over 75 rarely need a PSA test, unless they have a high risk for a Prostate Cancer such as:

    (a).   You have a family history of a prostate cancer, especially in a close relative such as a parent or siblings.

    (b).   Your relatives got Prostate Cancer before the age 60 or died from it before the age

75. These early cancer are more likely to grow faster.

(c).   If you have the above risks, you may want to ask your doctor about getting the PSA test before age 50.

(d).   Young women with an abnormal Pap-smear test **don't always need to be treated right away**. In the past, doctors thought that abnormal Pap-smear tests always meant Cervical Cancer. But now we know that isn't so. Minor abnormalities usually don't turn into cancer. Most go away on their own in a year or two, without any treatment.

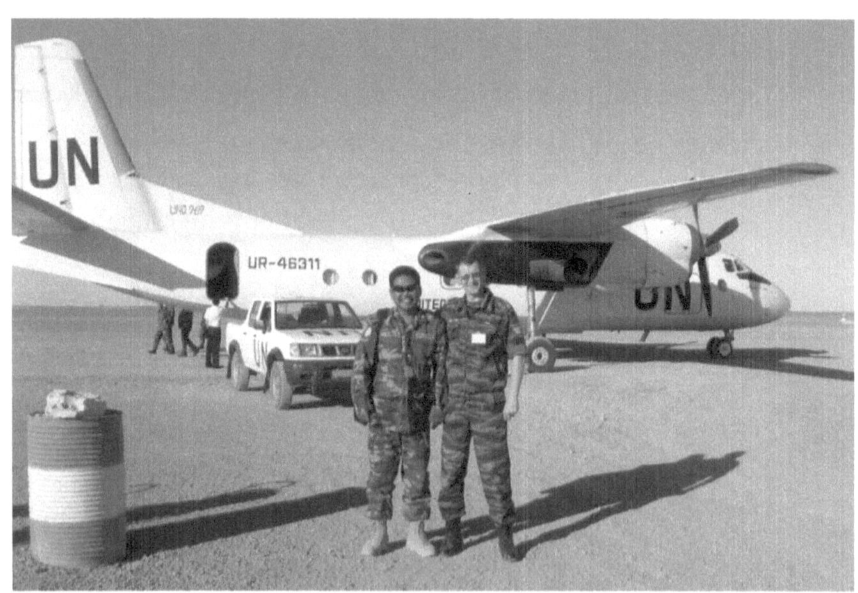

Picture-6: Another Mode of Transport in the Sahara Desert - With A Russian Colleague.

CHAPTER 6

THE COMMON COMPLAINT AND TREATMENT

A. BACK-PAIN

'It is much more important to know what sort of a patient has a disease than what sort of a disease a patient has.'

- *William Osler*

Some of the most common complaints at the General Practitioner's clinics (GPs), or commonly called the Private Clinics in Malaysia are:

1.   Acute Upper Respiratory Tract Infections (URTIs).
2.   Headaches, Migraines, Dizzy spells, Vertigos or Fainting attacks.
3.   Back pain.
4.   Abdominal problems.

I will use three of these most common complaints i.e. Backpain, Headaches and Acute Upper Respiratory Infections (URTIs), and in that particular order to explain the differences between the treatment that we are getting from the government hospitals and the private sectors.

Back Pain

Back pain or Backache are the same complaints. I will use both of these terms interchangeably so that we are familiar with both of them. As I have mentioned earlier, back pain is one of the most common complaints at the GP's clinic in Malaysia. Since backache is very crucial to this book in order for me to explain my theory of 'Simple Medicine- 3 Minutes Management (SM-3MM)', I will write a great deal about this complaint of backache.

When I was working with the Military as a medical doctor from 1996 to 2009, back pain was also one of the most common complaints that the military personnel came to our clinics. We could easily have hundreds if not thousands of patients with **chronic back pain.**

I was not surprised at all with this high number of patients with the back pain in the military. The nature of their work and their training involved many strenuous physical activities such as combat training, long distance marching, running, jungle trekking, mountain climbing, obstacle courses and parachute jumping while carrying heavy military equipment behind their back at all time.

They were also required to play all sort of dangerous sports such as rugby, football and hockey. These activities have high risks of injuries to the military personnel including the back injuries.

When I left the military and opened up my own private clinics in 2009, I was very surprised to see that there were more civilian patients who complained of back pain compared to the military personnel. I can understand the military personnel that had the back pain, but to have more patients that complained of the back pain from the office workers was very puzzling and baffling.

The treatment for the back pain at the government hospitals or the military hospitals were very straightforward. **In most cases, they were treated conservatively with pain-killers or muscle relaxants, massage creams, medicated plasters or with lumbar or cervical supports.**

In the military medical services during the time that I was there, I would confidently say that 99.9% of the patients with the back pain were treated conservatively as mentioned above. In fact, as far as I could remember, none of the patients had ever received any other form of treatment such as the steroid injections or back surgeries.

Some of the patients might be accepted for the physiotherapy treatment. As they were very busy, they did not just want to accept everybody for their physiotherapy treatment. They wanted to reserve their treatment for more severe cases or for patients that need to be rehabilitated to regain their muscle or joint functions.

I will give a few examples of the actual cases that we had when I was there and how the military doctors treated these cases. I would also write about other back pain cases that were treated at the government and private hospitals.

<u>Case No. 13</u>
Captain A,
A Fighter Jet Pilot,
RMAF.

Captain A was a young fighter jet pilot in his late 20s working with The Royal Malaysian Air Force (RMAF). One day he was flying as a passenger in a small transport plane going to one of the RMAF Bases. Unfortunately, the plane developed technical problems and crashed.

In the 5 years that I was serving in the RMAF (the other 9 years of my services were in the Army and Navy), I was involved as a member of the Board of Inquiry (BOI) in 5 aircraft crashes. All 11 personnel on-board these aircrafts were killed. The aircrafts involved were:

1.   3 x Pilatus PC-7 Training Jets.
2.   1 x Hawk Light Attack Jet.
3.   1 x Nuri Helicopter.

Luckily this time, all the pilots and passengers survived the crash. However, Captain A complained of a very severe back pain. Even though no military hospitals at that time had MRI machines, but they had special budgets for the pilots to do urgent tests at any of the private hospitals if necessary. They had these budgets so that if their pilots require any urgent tests or treatment, they would get them fast.

Before I write further, I would just like to explain a little bit more here about the fighter pilots. They are a different type of people, definitely not like us the ordinary people. They are leaders, very motivated, confident, extrovert, possess self-control, opportunistic, persistent, risk takers, self-aware and they do not accept the word 'cannot'. If you remember watching Tom Cruise in the *Top Gun (1986)*, then that Tom Cruise is them.

They accept that their work is very dangerous. They also accept that they can die at any time from a very minor mistake. Therefore, they are not the type of people who would worry about having headaches, migraines, dizzy spells, vertigos, heartburn, chest pain or back pain. They are the type of people who would do exercise every day to keep their bodies super fit so that they can do the Anti-G Straining Manoeuvre (AGSM) to sustain the persistent high G-Force during flying.

Anyway, the MRI results showed that he did not have any acute traumas such as the nerves impingement, fractured bones or any other injuries to his back. Unfortunately he was found to have Prolapsed of Inter-vertebral Discs (PIDs) or Slipped Discs at four different levels of his Lumbar Vertebra. These Slipped discs could have been an accidental finding, meaning that they could have been there even before the crash. They were not caused by the crash.

Since he did not have any acute injuries to his back, and he completely recovered from his back pain, our Military Orthopaedic Consultant sent him back to his Aviation Medical Doctors. They had a centre or head office called the Institute of Aviation Medicine (IAM) at the RMAF Subang, with no further action to be taken.

However, his case was taken over by one of the senior Aviation Medical Doctors at the IAM, whom we will call Lt Col (Dr) C. He was a very strict doctor. According to the regulations, a fighter pilot with PIDs or Slipped Discs are not allowed to fly a fast jet because in flying a fast jet, they will be subjected to a phenomenon called a high G-Force. This high G-Force will act directly along the backbone. In theory, pilots with PIDs or Slipped Discs will have the risks of having their problems worsened by flying in a high G-Force jet.

So Lt Col (Dr) C immediately suggested a Medical Board to be convened for Captain A. Eventually the medical board decided to downgrade his medical status from the best form i.e. *Forwards Everywhere (FE)*, which meant that he was fit for employment in full combatant duties (in any area) in any part of the world including flying a fighter jet, to the lowest form i.e. *Bases Everywhere (BE)*, which meant that he was only allowed to do limited ground duties and was confined to office work. It also meant that his flying career was finished.

Both Captain A and Lt. Col. (Dr) C went to the same Royal Military College (RMC) as I did. Both of them were my seniors. During our schooldays, Captain A used to be a rank holder (a prefect in normal school), a president for one of the biggest student societies and very active in sports and in everything else. He was the type of person who did not mind working 24 hours a day even though he was only required to work 8 hours a day, or would still manage to do his work even if he was not well.

Captain A protested the Medical Board decision. Yes, Captain A accepted that he had the PIDs or Slipped Discs, which was confirmed by the MRI scan. However, he never complained of any backache before the crash, or after the crash once his back pain due to the plane crash disappeared. His PIDs never interfered with his flying duties. The only reason it became an issue was because the doctors decided to do an MRI scan, which he never requested anyway. It soon involved the IAM's director and other officers as well, and the outcome was a bit complicated to explain here.

However, we could learn a few things from this case:

1. A person that was confirmed with having PIDs or Slipped Discs by an MRI scan at 4 different levels would not necessarily have any symptoms of back pain.

2. A person with confirmed Slipped Discs, who was previously involved in vigorous and strenuous physical activities i.e. military training for many years, would still have no back pain.

3. A person with confirmed Slipped Discs, who was previously involved in vigorous and strenuous physical activities for many years, and was flying fast jets with high-G force would still have no back pain.

4. A person with confirmed Slipped Discs, who was previously involved in vigorous and strenuous physical activities for many years, was flying fast jets with high-G force, and then was involved in a plane crash, would still have no back problems (he had no more back pain after the initial back pain due to the crash resolved).

5.   A fighter pilot with confirmed Slipped Discs, who was previously involved in vigorous and strenuous physical activities for many years, was flying fast jets with high-G force, and then was involved in a plane crash still did not end up with either the steroid injections or back surgeries. Whereas in a private sector, a patient who got his backache from sitting in air-conditioned office on a very comfortable office chair for a little too long would end up with 2 or 3 operations.

6.   A fighter pilot with confirmed Slipped Discs, who was previously involved in vigorous and strenuous physical activities for many years, was flying fast jets with high-G force, and then was involved in a plane crash **only had an MRI done once.** *That MRI scan did not alter the treatment that he was getting, but ruined his career for his whole life.* In contrast, a civilian patient with a backpain would require a regular MRI scans, sometimes once a year or even for every 6 months.

7.   The military Orthopaedic Consultants were only involved in a small part of this pilot's back pain problem. In fact, as what happen in most similar cases in the military, the orthopaedic surgeons would immediately discharge this patient from the orthopaedic department. They were not going to do any active treatment to this patient anymore, *not even a physiotherapy treatment.*

In general, the fighter pilots are supposed to have more back problems if compared to any other groups of people. They have to undergo vigorous and strenuous military training throughout their flying careers until they get to the top management posts. Their jet seats are very hard, unmoveable and very uncomfortable. The most important thing is that the high-G force during flying puts a heavy strain on their backbone.

However, they are the least likely people to complain of back pain to the doctors, especially to their aviation medical doctors. Why? Because they knew exactly what was going to happen. They would be treated conservatively as I have mentioned above, and they would be investigated for their back problems. If they were found to have

Slipped Discs, they would then be subjected to a medical board. Their physical status would be downgraded.

Once downgraded, they would lose two things, they would lose their seniority and their flying allowance. Because of that, they would have less chances of being promoted to higher ranks as well. Somehow, all these reasons would block whatever nerves that go to their brains that would make them complain not only for the back pain, but also for other complaints.

<u>Case No. 14</u>
Captain S,
A VIP's Helicopter Pilot.

Captain S started his flying career when he was in the Police Air Wing. He was already a fixed wing pilot or aeroplane when he was selected to do a basic flying training for helicopters in Australia in 1996. According to him, it costed the Malaysian Government about RM 1 million ringgit for each student pilot to complete the training at that time, and that was only for a basic training.

Unfortunately, during one of the flying lessons, he and his instructor crashed their helicopter. The instructor was teaching him the action that he was supposed to take if the engine suddenly stop. According to Captain S, all of a sudden the engine really stopped, and the helicopter just plummeted down to earth from about 1,000 feet high position at an almost a free fall speed.

The helicopter suffered a total loss. The instructor sustained a very bad back injuries, which made him having permanent paralysis of both of his lower limbs. Captain S suffered a severe back pain, with severe numbness in both legs and a bowel incontinence i.e. he cannot control his bladder.

Captain S was treated with a complete bed rest for almost 2 months, back braces, back manipulation and pain-killers or muscle relaxants. Luckily he fully recovered from the injuries, and completed his flying school. He suffered from 2 more crashes in his flying career, one in a fixed wing aircraft and the other one in another helicopter. Fortunately in both occasions he managed to save the aircrafts, with him suffering from non-life threatening injuries, including muscle and back pain.

He requested to leave the police service early. His jobs after leaving the police involved carrying VIPs. Now he is working with one of the most prominent Malaysian Businessman. May be his experiences in those 3 crashes and survived make these VIPs more confident in flying with him.

When I interviewed Captain S during one of his yearly pilot medical examination and asked his permission to include his story into this book, he told me that he rarely took the pain-killers for his back pain. One of the treatment that he thought helped him in controlling his back pain was a horse riding therapy. In this therapy, he was taught to ride a horse at a slow speed and control his body or back posture that gave him the least painful position with every step that the horse took.

We could learn a few things from Captain S's dangerous experiences here:

1.	Even a helicopter pilot that crashed from a 1,000 feet high position at an almost a free fall speed with a total loss of the helicopter and suffered a severe back pain with numbness in both of his lower limbs and uncontrolled bladder, was only treated conservatively with a bed rest, pain-killers or muscle relaxants, back supports and back manipulations.

2.	A helicopter pilot that was involved in 3 aircraft crashes with severe back pain did not end up with either a steroid injection or a back surgery. He did not even need to go for a long term physiotherapy treatment either.

3.	Even in a traumatic severe back pain patient like in this case, he was treated conservatively and fully recovered from his back injuries. In contrast in the private sectors, a non-traumatic back pain could end with a few steroid injections to their back or even a few back surgeries.

Case No. 15

Commandos A and B,
Grup Gerak Khas (GGK),
Malaysia.

One day I had to do a medical cover for a group of commandos who were doing their training in Hulu Terengganu. The scenario of their training was that they would fly from their camp in Malacca, and would arrive in Hulu Terengganu late in the evening. They would use the darkness to camouflage their arrival. They would then jump from the aircraft using the static parachutes (the round-shaped parachute) from a height of about 1,000 feet, pack their things, and walk for another 30 to 40 kms to the Kenyir Dam. They would then ambush the enemies who were supposed to be there.

During the jump, two of the commando personnel had their parachutes collided with each other. Both of the parachutes collapsed. Both of them fell to the ground at an almost free-fall speed. It happened not very far from where we, the medical personnel were standing. May be just about 30 to 40 meters away. I was shocked to see that happening in front of my eyes. We immediately picked up the stretchers and ran to get them.

Before I write further, I would just like to explain a little bit more here about our commandos. They are our no-nonsense military personnel. They are our most elite soldiers and highly trained for special operations.

They are mentally and physically very tough, smart, very determined, highly skilled people, resourceful, loyal, calm, discreet and many more. They are the type of soldiers that can be dropped into a jungle in their underwears and they can survive there for weeks or months. If you remember watching Arnold Schwarzenegger in the *Commando (1985)*, then that Arnold Schwarzenegger is them. Except that, their bodies and muscles are much smaller.

They need to keep their bodies super fit and they need to be prepared mentally for their dangerous training. They know that their jobs are very dangerous so they need to be very focused to their jobs or missions. They are not the type of people who would worry about having headaches, migraines, dizzy spells, vertigos, heartburns or back pain.

When we arrived at the scene, and while I was still recovering from the shock, we immediately asked whether they were okay or not. Almost immediately, they replied that they were okay and they wanted to continue with their training. Commando A tried to get up but immediately collapsed to the ground and tried again, but the same thing happened.

We immediately stopped him from getting up and placed him on the stretcher. We told him better not to move and get his back checked first. We could see straight away how frustrated he was, because he could not continue with the training.

The other guy, Commando B, was able to get up and move around, but he had a big swelling at one of his ankles. Definitely, he had sprained it badly, or it could be a fracture. We wanted to bring him to the hospital together with Commando A, but he refused. He pleaded with us to allow him to continue his training, which we reluctantly agreed.

He immediately put a simple **CREPE bandage** over his injured ankle, which usually cost about RM3 or RM4, (no proper, expensive ankle guard), wore his sock and put his boot on. He then joined his team and disappeared into the night and into the hills nearby, or rather mountains. This 30 to 40 km march to the Kenyir Dam was not along the main road. The march was through the jungles, with many hills and mountains along the way.

About 6 months later I got the Commando A's medical report. It said that from the x-rays and MRI scans, they diagnosed him with multiple cracked fracture of four of his lumbar vertebrae bones. As the fractures were stable, they treated him conservatively with the lumbar braces and transferred him to the military hospital in Malacca for further management. Because of his fractures, his physical status was advised to be downgraded to *Bases Everywhere* (BE) Permanent. He would be excused from doing any strenuous physical activities until he retires from the military.

As for the Commando B, since I did not get any medical report, I presumed that he was treated conservatively by his unit's medical personnel with pain-killers, massage creams, bandages etc. He might not even have any x-rays or MRIs done.

We could make a few observations about Commando A:

1. A person that fell down at an almost free-fall speed from a 1,000 feet high moving aircraft did not require any operations or steroid injections to treat his back pain.

2. Even a person that had multiple cracked fractures of his lumbar vertebras did not require any operations or steroid injections to treat his back problems.

3. Like in most cases of the back pain in the military, after everything including the medical board has been done, he will not require any physiotherapy treatment, pain-killers, orthopaedic reviews or hospital admissions for his back problem anymore.

The commandos are also the group of people that are supposed to have more back problems compared to any other groups of people. They are in the same group as the fighter pilots. They have to undergo vigorous physical training throughout their commando career. I would easily say that I would not even last for a few minutes if I were to join the commando training.

However, they are the least likely people to complain of back pain to the doctors, especially to their unit medical doctors. Why? Because they knew exactly what was going to happen.

They would be treated conservatively as I have mentioned above, and they would be investigated for their back problems. If they were found to have Slipped Discs, they would be subjected to a medical board. Their physical status would be downgraded.

Once downgraded, they would lose two things, they would lose their seniority and their commando's allowance. Because of that, they would have less chances of being promoted to higher ranks as well. Somehow, all these reasons block whatever nerves that go to their brains that would make them complain not only for the back pain, but also for other complaints.

<h1 style="text-align:center"><u>Case No. 16</u>
Corporal A,
An Infantryman turned to a Clerk.</h1>

I was posted to a camp in the East Coast as the Senior Medical Officer in 2000. Apart from having the regular medical staff, I also had a corporal, whom we will call Corporal A. He was initially an infantry soldier but involved in a very bad motorcycle accident many years before.

He suffered multiple injuries to most part of his body and it was a miracle that he survived the crash. His medical status was already downgraded to a *Bases Everywhere* (BE) Permanent, which meant that he was only allowed to do light duties at the bases. He was attached to my unit to do clerical jobs.

His injuries were so severe that he was bed-ridden at the hospital for quite some time. He suffered from multiple injuries including head injuries, back injuries and multiple fractures of his long bones i.e. bones in the upper and lower limbs. When I met him, his injuries were already healed. He did not need any more treatment or medication.

Usually by this time, most hospitals would discharge their patients, as there will not be any more active treatment. However, his hospital insisted on seeing him once a year, may be they just wanted to see this miracle guy who was not supposed to survive his injuries.

If you see him walking, you can see that he was slightly limping. He had some limited movements at several joints of the upper limbs and lower limbs.

Apart from that, he was well and healthy. He could move around easily. He could ride his motorcycle to come to work or go back home, and he had a good appetite. He had no more pain and he did not need to take any medication, which means that he did not need anymore doctor's management. He did not need to attend any physiotherapy treatment either. He was a free man.

We could make a few observations from this case:

1. He was treated conservatively for most of his injuries. There were no operations done for his head injuries and back injuries. Even

his fractured bones were treated conservatively with the *Plaster of Paris (POP)* casts. Why? Because, as in a lot of cases, giving minimal treatment and allowing the body to heal itself gives a better outcome compared to giving active or invasive treatment.

2.   Even people with severe back injuries and fractured long bones did not need pain-killers, did not take any supplement like calcium and did not require any physiotherapy treatment.

3.   The government hospital did not order any repeat or new x-rays or MRIs for his head injuries, back injuries or for his fractured bones. They believed that his injuries had stabilised and did not need any more monitoring.

<u>Case No. 17</u>
Patient C,
A Housewife.

Patient C, one of my relatives, was a 69 years old woman. In general, she was healthy except that she had been complaining of a back pain for more than 15 years. When she bent over, we could see that her backbone looked like a letter S.

She had a severe scoliosis (abnormal lateral curvature of the spine) and a slight kyphosis (excessive outward curvature of the spine, causing hunching of the back) due to her osteoporosis, which caused her to have multiple levels of Prolapsed of the Intervertebral Discs (PIDs) or Slipped Discs. She was diagnosed as having Osteoporosis, Degenerative Scoliosis and Kyphosis with multiple levels of PIDs.

She was started on the Hormone Replacement Therapy (HRT) many years before. This would help to slow the rate of bone loss, as well as relieving the symptoms of menopause by restoring the oestrogen levels. However, she decided not to continue the treatment because she did not want to have any menstrual bleeding anymore.

She also refused to take the bisphosphonates medicine to prevent the loss of bone density, as it could cause irritation to the oesophagus and cause stomach pain and make her gastritis worse. She used the lumbar support intermittently, as it was not comfortable to wear for a long period.

Because of the above reasons and because of the progress of the disease, her back pain was getting worse. The pain could become worse when standing or walking for a long time, or doing some of the household chores. When we did a repeat of her back x-rays we could really see that the curvatures of her back bone and the prolapsed discs were getting worse.

We then brought her to one of the Teaching Hospitals or Medical Schools to see the consultant orthopaedic surgeon there. I was thinking at that time that surely the orthopaedic surgeon would order an urgent MRI scan, and would immediately advise her to go for an operation to correct her back bones.

At the hospital, the consultant orthopaedic surgeon who was also a Professor ordered a new set of back x-rays. He compared the new ones with the old ones. He then gave Patient A two options. The first option was to treat the problem conservatively with pain-killers, lumbar support, massage creams etc., as Patient A had no problems in looking after herself. He also advised her not to do any physical activities that would aggravate the back pain.

The second option was to go for a back surgery, but it could have its own complications such as nerve injuries with paralysis of the lower limbs, wound infections or even death.

Since Patient A was not keen on any operations, she happily accepted the first option. That was the only time she was seen by an orthopaedic surgeon (the first and only time by a specialist in her whole life).

From this case, we could make a few observations:

1.   A patient who used to have a straight backbone but deteriorated to look like a letter S and became 1 foot shorter still did not necessarily need an operation to correct her back problems.

2.   Even with a severe scoliosis and the backbone that looked like a letter S, MRI test is not necessary, because it did not necessarily change the management.

3.   Even in an old woman with Hypertension, she was treated with a strong pain-killer for her back pain by the Professor.

Case No. 18
Patient B,
A Project Engineer.

Patient B was a 44 years old man. He worked with an Oil and Gas (O&G) Company for many years. One of his job requirements was to entertain the staff from a big national oil company that they were getting contracts from. Apparently trying to make somebody else happy was very stressful.

About 10 years ago, he started complaining of neck pain with numbness of both of his upper limbs. As the pain and numbness were getting more and more serious, he decided to see one of the consultant orthopaedic surgeons at one of the private hospitals there. The MRIs of the neck showed that he had Prolapsed of the Intervertebral Discs (PIDs) or Slipped Discs at 3 different levels of his cervical bones.

He was then advised to go for an urgent operation to correct his slipped discs. The operation would cost about RM50,000.00 per level. His company at that time was doing well and would not have any problems to pay for his operation.

While being admitted to the hospital for the operation, the orthopaedic surgeon explained to him about the many complications that could happen during the operation. One of them was to lose the voice, or to wake up with a different voice.

He was so shocked hearing that that he canceled the admission, refused the operation and went back home. That was about 7 or 8 years ago. Now magically his neck pain and numbness in his upper limbs have disappeared, without any operations done or taking any medication.

Now he rarely talks about it or complains of the neck pain anymore. The fact that he is afraid of the operation block whatever nerves that go to the brain that would make him complain of having a neck pain.

<u>Case No. 19</u>
Lieutenant Colonel (Lt Col) A,
A United Nations' colleague.

During one of my United Nations' missions, I became close to one of the senior officers from a South American country. We became so close that we could talk about everything. Previously he had a very severe back problems. Since his work in his country involved standing for a long period of time, the back pain became an issue because it interfered with his work.

Like many other South American people, he had many relatives in the US. He managed to arrange for a back surgery to be done there with the help of his relatives who were living in the US. Unfortunately, his back pain came back one month after the expensive operation done in the US.

Then he realised that even though he was successful in his career, his personal life was miserable. He was divorced three times. Many of his wives and kids were suing him for the alimony and for child support. Because of that, he was always stressed.

Since even the expensive back surgery done in the US did not solve his back problems, he started doing something else for his back problem. Initially he started doing back exercises to make his back muscles stronger. Then he started jogging. Even though initially the jogging caused discomfort at his back, like Prof. Dr A in Case No. 8 above, he persistently continued with his running activities. At the same time, he tried to solve all his personal issues.

When I met him during that mission, he never complained of any back pain at all. He was also the only military personnel that jogged every day without fail for almost 6 months that we were there.

<u>Case No. 20</u>
Multiple Soldiers,
Malaysia.

Our military personnel are divided into 2 different groups, officers and non-officers. The non-officers usually retire early. They could retire after 21 or 22 years of service. Their services started the moment they joined the military. This means that their training is also included as their service years.

If they started their training at the age of 18, they could retire at the age of 39 or 40 years old. Since being a normal, non-officer military personnel involve a lot of physical training and activities, they would have many back problems or joint problems when they are in their 30s. It is the same with the sportsmen or footballers, by 30 years old they are already old.

At a certain time or age, some of these soldiers knew that they were not going to be promoted anymore. They were stuck with the low ranks like corporals or sergeants. Because of these, they were still required to undergo the tough training or the strenuous physical activities like the young soldiers needed to do. Some of them thought that enough was enough. They usually came to us the military doctors with specific complaints, most commonly with the back pain.

We need to solve their problems, otherwise they would cause problems at their respective units. However, our orthopaedic surgeons usually did not want to just accept anybody with a simple back pain. To them they were wasting their time, because they were not going to give any active treatment like surgeries to these soldiers.

If you remember Captain A and Commando A above, in both cases our orthopaedic surgeon's contribution was purely administrative. What they need to do was to order MRI scans to confirm whether there were any abnormalities or not. The MRIs were reported by other doctors anyway i.e. the Radiologists. Whether there were Slipped Discs or not, what they need to do was to follow whatever the MRI reports were given by the Radiologists.

They would then recommend whether a medical board should be convened, based on that MRI report. Immediately after the report, they would discharge the patients back to their respective doctors. The problem was we needed that report, usually on a piece of paper, to convene the medical board.

Therefore, when we referred these soldiers to them we needed to make the letters sound more dramatic. Usually we would write: *'Dear Sir. Thank you for accepting this 35 years old army personnel.*

He had been complaining of a back pain for the past 10 years due to a fall during a jungle exercise. His back pain has become more frequent and more severe for the past 3 years and unbearable for the past 6 months. He finds it very difficult to follow his unit's activities...'. and so on. The true story was not that far from this dramatized one.

Even with this dramatic referral letter, the orthopaedic surgeons would still give us an appointment in 3 to 6 months' time. Then he would order an MRI scan, which would take another 3 to 6 months, and we have to wait another few months for that one piece of medical report.

How different this scenario is with the private sectors. A patient with a 4 days history of a back pain without any history of trauma would be seen immediately, not only by the orthopaedic surgeon, but by the spine surgeon (a sub-specialist from the orthopaedic surgeon). Sometimes the MRI would be done on the same day, and many would end up with back surgeries, like what happened to Mr C in Case No. 10 above. Unfortunately the surgery did not resolve his problem, but left him paralysed for life.

If these soldiers' MRI reports were normal, then bad luck, they will not be excused from any of the physical exercises or training. If the MRI reports confirmed that they had Slipped Discs, then medical boards would be convened for them. Their physical status would be downgraded. They would be excused from any physical exercises or training, and assigned to desk jobs.

Usually after we had the medical boards done for these soldiers with Slipped Discs, we will not have to treat their problems anymore. They do not need any pain-killers, other medicine or the physiotherapy treatment, except in a small number of cases. They would be happy doing desk jobs at their units.

However, other problems arose. Since these soldiers' medical status were downgraded and they were assigned to desk jobs, other soldiers needed to do more physical works at their respective units. Usually the other soldiers would be complaining that they saw these personnel doing heavy work outside their camp (after working hours) such as operating a food stall or doing other second jobs with no problems. However, they could not do any physical activities during their actual work in their respective camps.

Usually, we needed to explain to the other soldiers that we decided based on the MRI's findings. If it was confirmed that they had slipped discs in the MRIs, then the rules said that their physical status should be downgraded.

We could make a few observations about these soldiers:

1.	Even a person that had a long history of back pain did not require any active treatment for his back pain such as the steroid injection or back surgery.

2.	A person that had Slipped Discs would not have back pain if they liked what they were doing. Usually these soldiers would start a second job outside their working hours like opening a restaurant, in preparation for them to leave the military service.

3.	Like in most cases of the back pain in the Military, after everything have been done including the medical boards, they did not require any pain-killers, physiotherapy treatment, orthopaedic reviews or hospital admissions for their back problems.

None of our military personnel with the back pain or slipped discs during my time in the military service died, became paralysed or had other bad complications from their back problems. In fact, most of them did not have as frequent an attack of back pain as my civilian patients. Capt A as in the Case No. 13 above is a 2-star General now, with no complaint of back pain at all.

CHAPTER 7

THE COMMON COMPLAINT AND TREATMENT

B. HEADACHES, MIGRAINES, DIZZY SPELLS, VERTIGOS AND FAINTING ATTACKS

'What you are thinking is what you're becoming'.

-        *Anonymous*

Another common complaint at the GPs' clinics is a headache, or something similar to the headache such as a dizzy spell, a vertigo or a fainting attack. Again many of the patients at my private clinics either request to see a neurologist or a neurosurgeon for a further treatment of their problems, or end up with the CT-scans or MRIs done, or both.

Case No. 21
Ms A,
A 22 y.o Malay Woman.

Once at a clinic, Ms A was brought in unconscious. After checking all the vital signs, her ABCs (Airways, Breathing and Circulations) and her Central and Peripheral Nervous Systems, I decided to just let her rest since all the vital signs and the nervous systems were normal.

At the same time, we were trying to contact her relatives by using whatever information that we could get from her wallet. I was quite busy at that time that I did not realise Ms A had remained unconscious for almost 8 hours.

Fortunately, she regained her consciousness. Even though initially she was a bit groggy, she returned to her normal self not long after that and I was able to take a full history from her. Apparently, she had been complaining of headaches, dizzy spells and fainting attacks for the past several years.

She was admitted to a few private hospitals on many occasions. They have checked almost everything, including the blood and urine tests, x-rays, ECGs, ultra-sounds, the EEGs and MRIs of the brain, but everything was normal. She was not even on any long-term medication.

We could learn a few things from this case:

1.   A patient that had headaches, dizzy spells and fainted for 8 hours still could not have any serious medical problems.

2.   A patient that had headaches, dizzy spells and fainted for 8 hours did not have any abnormalities with her blood and urine tests, x-rays, ECGs, ultra-sounds, EEGs or MRI scans.

3.   A patient that had headaches, dizzy spells and fainted for 8 hours was not given any medication either to treat her conditions or to prevent her from having the fainting attacks.

4.   A patient that had headaches, dizzy spells and fainted for 8 hours did not need any medication or intravenous fluids even in the acute attack. I did not give her anything, not even a Paracetamol tablet, except letting her rest in bed.

5.   A patient that had headaches, dizzy spells and fainted for 8 hours did not get any complications from her fainting attack or from her unconsciousness.

Cost Of Admitting Patients To The Hospital

Usually at the hospitals, once an unconscious patient is admitted, they have to do many tests and giving treatment according to their Standard Operating Procedures (SOPs). They have to check all the vital signs, monitor the pulse rate, monitor the heart, give oxygen and monitor the oxygen concentration, do some routine blood and urine tests, chest x-ray and many more. They would also set the intravenous fluid lines so that if they need to give any intravenous drug injections urgently they already have the lines or veins open.

They do all these monitoring and investigations so that they do not miss anything important. Most of the time they also need to do other specific tests as well, for e.g. x-rays for the other parts of the body, ultrasounds, MRIs or CT-scans. All these tests cost a lot of money even in the government hospitals and would cost much more in the private hospitals. That is why sometimes the hospital bill could run into hundreds of thousands of ringgit, even though the patients do not survive the ordeal.

I can still remember in 2000 when I just joined a medical unit in the east coast of Peninsular Malaysia, my corporal came to me in distress. She told me that one of her relatives was involved in a road traffic accident. He suffered serious injuries and they took him to the nearest private hospital. The doctors there did an emergency surgery to try to save him, but he succumbed to his injuries.

The bill came up to about RM120,000.00 and they did not have that much money to pay to the hospital. This case happened 20 years ago. It should cost much more now for a similar case. In the US they have to do more tests and investigations than what we do in Malaysia so that if anything goes wrong (defensive medicine), they could defend themselves from any litigation process. That is why the health care costs much more in the US, which could run into millions of dollars for each patient.

Sometimes, we purposely do a few procedures or treatment to the patients to show to the relatives that we are doing something and are treating the patients. We do that for the sake of the relatives to reduce their anxieties or angers, not for the patients. I could still remember one late night during my internship when we had a middle-aged man brought in for a Road Traffic Accident (RTA). Yes, bad cases always happen at night when many of the doctors have gone home. He had a low Glasgow Coma Scale (GCS) of 8/15, and slowly dropping.

The Glasgow Coma Scale or GCS is a simple method that we use to assess any patients that has head injuries. In normal people, the GCS would be 15/15. The lowest is 3/15, which means the patient is dead. At GCS of 8/15, and dropping meant that he was not in a good shape. His Haemoglobin level that the A&E doctors checked was very low, which suggested that he had an internal bleeding. They had already ordered bloods for possible blood transfusion.

When they transferred this patient to us from the surgical team at the A&E ward, both of his pupils were already fixed and dilated. It meant that he was already brain dead. Therefore, we decided not to do any active managements for him. The relatives at this time were in distressed, crying and running around to make calls to other relatives or hugging with each other.

Suddenly the head of the surgical department appeared as he was doing a late night ward round. He called us into a room and asked us to just pretend doing something to the patient including giving the blood transfusion since we already had the blood ready, so that the relatives thought that we were doing everything we could to save their father's life. After doing all those things then would we explain the real situation to the relatives.

<u>Case No. 22</u>
Private A,
A mid-30s soldier.

I was posted to a camp in Kelantan as the Senior Medical Officer in 2000 i.e. I would be the officer in-charge there. The first thing that I found out was that, apart from the regular medical staff that I had, I also had one infantry guy attached to the clinic. He had had a medical board done for a migraine. His medical status was downgraded to *BE Permanent*.

As he cannot cope with working in an infantry unit, he was attached to my clinic to do odd jobs. Every day I noticed that he spent only about 30 minutes doing productive works like sweeping the floor, a little bit of gardening or a few other minor jobs. The rest of the day, he will be resting in his room or resting at the gazebo and not doing anything. He had been doing this for many years since before I came to this clinic.

For me as a young military officer at that time, that was not fair. Since he was collecting his salary, then he should have been doing much more than that. Therefore, I told my Staff Sergeant to tell him that since I found him to be in a good health with a nice, fit body, I wanted him to be sent back to his former unit. I knew that if he were sent to his former unit, he would be asked to do much more work even though he had a medical board done.

Then suddenly he started having his migraine attack again and very frequently on top of that. Whenever he was having his attack, he would be lying on the floor holding his head with both of his hands crying, and he would regularly bang his head either to the cement floor or to the cement wall. This attack would last for a few hours each time. Even as a doctor, it was very scary to look at him during the attacks. Everything was real and very dramatic.

After a few attacks, I let him know that I had changed my mind. He could stay at my clinic as long as he liked. As if by magic, his attacks were getting less and less in frequency and severity. The attacks were quicker to recover too.

Initially I thought of doing a few new blood tests, or order a new skull x-ray or referred for a new MRI scan. It could be a new medical problem in his brain. However, since his attack was getting lesser, I decided not to do anything. I did not give him any medication during the attack, not even a paracetamol tablet.

We could make a few comments from this case:

1.   A patient that had a severe headache, and had to bang his head to the cement walls for a few hours still would not have any medical problems. *Migraine is a diagnosis by exclusion.* If somebody has regular headaches but all the tests are normal, then we would diagnose him or her as having a migraine. There is no test that could confirm a patient is suffering from a migraine.

2.   A patient that had a severe headache, and had to bang his head to the cement walls for a few hours did not need any medication or intravenous fluid even in the acute attack. I did not give him anything, not even a paracetamol tablet. Usually in that situation the patient did not like to take anything orally, and when I was a young doctor I did not like to just inject everybody with a strong pain-killer either. I just let him rest on the floor.

3.   Anything that the patient does not like could trigger the migraine attack.

<u>Case No. 23</u>
Motorcyclist A,
A young Malay guy (in his 20s).

One late night when I was on-call during my houseman year, I had a patient whom we will call Motorcyclist A. Since General Surgery was my first posting during my houseman-ship, I must have started working for only 1 or 2 months earlier, not having much of an experience.

Anyway, this motorcyclist A was brought into the emergency ward from the Accident and Emergency Department. It meant that the A&E doctors had passed over this patient to my surgical team. They had found that Motorcyclist A did not have any bone fractures or any major internal injuries. However, he had a large laceration wound starting from his left eyebrow, extending up to the scalp and end at the back of his head. His wound could easily be 12 inches long. He also had a Glasgow Coma Scale (GCS) of 13/15.

Again, in a normal people the GCS would be 15/15. The lowest is 3/15, which means the patient is dead. Therefore, at GCS of 13/15, this motorcyclist A was in delirium, shouting at everybody, or at nobody off and on without any reasons. Sometimes he was lying there quietly but suddenly he would wake up and trying to jump out from the bed. You could not make a conversation with him, or ask him to calm down. Because of that, we had to tie both of his hands and feet to the bed.

Since his GCS was 13/15, it was not low enough to warrant for an urgent CT-Scan of the brain. Somehow, most of the bad cases always took place late at night when all the specialists were at home, so we had to call our on-call specialist to request for an urgent CT-scan. Otherwise, the radiology department would refuse to do that. (Yes, our radiology department refused to do an urgent CT-scan even on a patient with a 12 inch-long scalp laceration wound and a GCS of 13/15, unless our consultant requested for it). The on-call specialist had to come to the emergency ward, signed the CT-scan form, and went back home.

The CT-scan came back as normal, which meant that there were no injuries in the brain that require any further action. We decided to close his laceration wound with a local anaesthesia. It was not advisable to do it under a General Anaesthesia since he was delirious and with a GCS of 13/15.

As the houseman on-call, I had to close his laceration wound. That was the most difficult wound that I had to do in my whole life. Every time I inserted the needle into his skin, he would be screaming and struggling to get away from me. I had to ask the nurses to pin him down so that I could finish the job. Every stitch was a big struggle to do.

It took me at least 4 to 5 hours to close the wound from the back of the head until the hairline of the forehead. Initially I wanted to finish the job and close the entire wound until his left eyebrow. However, since it was very difficult to do that, I left the rest of the wound to the plastic department to finish it. Usually they were the one that would close the wound on the face.

After a few days in the ward, his GCS scores returned to normal to 15/15. We discharged him well except a big wound on the scalp. Miraculously he did not have any other injuries or complications from the accident.

We could learn a few things from this case:

1.	A person that had a head injury due to a high impact force that caused him to have a big laceration wound on the head and reduced his GCS score to 13/15 would still have no brain injuries. We discharged him from the ward with a simple pain-killer.

2.	If you fall down and complain of a headache which persist, do not worry. If you can see, talk, walk and move around, it means that you have a GCS of 15/15. Another major signs for a normal functioning brain are eating and the absence of vomiting. If you can eat and does not vomit, then you don't need to do any skull x-ray or even a CT-scan or an MRI-test to check your brain. I had on many occasions patients insisted of going for a CT scan or an MRI for the above problems.

<u>Case No. 24</u>
Ms B (in late 20s),
A Young Chinese Woman.

When I left the Military Services in 2009, I opened up one of my clinics in a new, big development project in Kuala Lumpur. The clinic was in a shopping complex, which was surrounded by many big and tall office buildings, condominiums and hotels. Now the clinic has moved to a new building nearby.

There were many multi-national companies as well as big Malaysian companies there. So most of our patients were office workers. The majority of them were professionals like the IT consultants, programmers, accountants, auditors, white-collar officers and so on. On many occasions, they called me to come to their offices because somebody had fainted or had fallen unconscious.

One of these patients who fainted or fell unconscious was Ms B, a woman in her late 20s. It happened a few times. Usually I would go up and see her at the office. If I found that her condition was not that serious, I would ask her to be brought down to the clinic, either by a wheelchair or by a stretcher.

Ms B's symptoms were usually more significant than the other patients. She would complain of headaches, dizzy spells, losing consciousness, left-sided chest discomfort, sweating and shortness of breath. These symptoms were as if she was having a heart attack. Even though I believed that it would be very rare for a young lady who was not menopausal to have a heart attack. Unless that woman had long-standing medical problems such as diabetes or hypertension.

What I remember most about her was that her pulse rate was very fast, about 150 to 160 beats per minute (bpm). Other tests like the blood pressure, blood sugar and ECG were normal. These fast heart rates could be very dangerous. It could lead to a cardiac arrest. Usually I would immediately refer her to one of the big private hospitals nearby.

When I saw her later, she told me that she was thoroughly examined at the private hospitals for a few times. The tests done included the blood and urine tests, x-rays, stress test, echocardiography for the heart, MRIs for the brain and many more. However, all these tests were normal.

When I asked her further questions, she admitted to having many personal and work problems. At work, usually she could not meet the target that she was supposed to achieve. Eventually she resigned from her job and got a less stressful job.

We could learn a few things from this case:

1. It is very uncommon or rare to have a young adult woman to suddenly have major medical problems. In this case even in somebody with many significant signs and symptoms like a severe headache, dizzy spells, a left-sided chest pain, sweating, fast heart rates and falling unconscious were found to have normal test results with no medical issues.

2. In most cases that involved young patients i.e. less than 50 years old for a woman and less than 40 years old for a man, most of the tests done at the hospitals would be normal and the doctors could not give a definite diagnosis. In these cases, the causes were more likely to be stress related, either personal or work related, or both.

<u>Case No. 25</u>
Ms C, D and E,
Young Malaysian Ladies.

Somehow, I noticed that most people that complain of frequent headaches, migraines, dizzy spells, vertigo or fainting attacks were young or middle-aged women. These could be due to the nature of the women, who like to think about everything until everything becomes their problems. The life of modern women nowadays are also much more complicated than the life of the traditional women before.

Both my grandmother and my mother are homemakers. Their main jobs are to look after the kids and do household chores. I remember when I was young, Saturday evenings were their movie times. They would make sure that all the household chores were finished before 3.00pm just before the Hindi or Tamil movies started on TV3. Usually they would watch the movies with a few neighbours. The most interesting part was that they would spend another few hours after the movies to discuss and comment among themselves regarding the movies that they just watched.

Modern women usually need to work, look after their children, take care of the family especially the financial burden, do household chores, take care of their parents and many more. Whereas for the husbands most of them do not have to worry as many problems as the wives do. There are some husbands who do not even have any jobs. They become dependent on their wives for everything. Sometimes they are not doing anything for the whole day, but still expect their wives to take care of all their needs.

Ms C was a young Chinese lady in her mid-20s. She had been complaining of headaches, dizzy spells, vertigo and fainting attacks for many years. She had had MRIs done on two different occasions. Both were normal. But she still came to my clinic worrying about her problems and thought of doing other tests for her problems.

Ms D was a first year Malay medical student. Her parents divorced many years before and her mother became a single parent. Apart from the usual headaches and dizzy spells, she also complained of many other non-specific symptoms. She had both MRI and CT-scan done for her brain, but both were normal.

Ms E was a young mother of two in her mid-20s. She was working in a private sector but could not cope with her work. She was admitted to the private hospitals on a few occasions because of the same complaints i.e. headaches, migraines, dizzy spells and fainting attacks. All the investigations done which include the MRIs were normal. Because of her regular sick-leaves and her medical bills, her company refused to let her go for any more expensive investigations or procedures at the hospital.

Ms E came to me requesting for her to be referred to a government hospital for another MRI scan. She was still convinced that there was something wrong with her body, especially the brain that could not be detected by the previous private hospitals.

I have so many patients with similar problems as above. In fact, I swear that I had a few patients who had done almost all the tests and procedures that were available at the hospitals. They have had the MRIs or CT scans or both for their headaches, endoscopy and colonoscopy done for their gastritis, angiograms for their left-sided chest pain, spine surgeries for their slipped discs and yet they come with more complaints. These procedures did not include the normal tests like the blood and urine tests, x-rays or ultra-sounds.

Usually in these cases, I would try to convince them that they should stop doing any more tests or procedures. In fact, they should stop from going to any hospitals. They should stop worrying about their health and should start enjoying their lives instead.

<u>Case No. 26</u>
Mr E,

A Hospital Staff.

When I was working in the government or military hospitals, we rarely admit patients who had headaches or with Acute Upper Respiratory Tract Infections (URTIs). Most of the time we would just treat them with simple medication and asked them to come back if necessary. The reason we did not want to admit them was because these two medical problems rarely cause any bad or significant complications.

One day when I was working in the medical department of this government hospital, one of the hospital staff, Mr E was admitted to our medical ward for a headache. The medical wards at any hospitals are usually very busy 24 hours a day, 7 days a week. Patients in bad conditions could be admitted at any time of the day.

Once I have admitted (we call it clerk-in) Mr E, I passed him to the medical officer in-charge of the ward for further managements. This medical officer was a difficult doctor. From my examination, he did not have any other significant signs and symptoms except the headache.

After looking at the file, he immediately called the A&E doctor who admitted the patient and scolded him. He was very angry because the A&E doctor admitted a patient with a simple diagnosis. For him this was an unnecessary hospital admission.

I remembered this case clearly. Mr E was having a severe headache. He was restless, sitting on the bed and holding his head constantly. He could not even lie down or go to sleep. As usual for any patient that we admit to the ward, we needed to do a set of blood and urine tests, ECG, CXR and Skull X-ray on Mr A.

All the tests came back as normal. However, Mr A was still restless throughout the night and could not sleep until the next day. We treated him with pain-killers and kept monitoring his vital signs.

The next day, somehow Mr A's headache was completely gone. He did not have any complications or bad side effects from the headache. This is what usually happen with a headache. Even though the bad complications that a patient could have from a headache like what we read in the newspapers could happen, in general these are very rare. That is the reason why the government hospitals do not just want to admit any patients with a simple headache. For them they are wasting the hospital's resources.

<u>**Case No. 27**</u>
Student A,
Dublin, Ireland.

Once when I was a student in Dublin, Ireland in the 1990s, a friend had a severe headache in the middle of the night. In Ireland, as in the UK you cannot simply go to their Emergency Departments without any referral letters from your doctor.

You need to contact your General Practitioner (GP) first. Your GP will advise you what action should be taken next. After listening to his complaint, his doctor decided to see him at his house. We call this a house visit. Their aim was not to send any patient to the Emergency Department unnecessarily.

After doing a few examinations, the doctor diagnosed him as having a simple headache. He gave him a few paracetamol tablets and charged him £40 (about RM220.00, and they were still using the Irish pound at that time instead of the euro) for the visit.

To spend £40 for a student during that time was a lot of money. He was very upset with the charges and thought that he should have just taken the paracetamol tablets first before calling his GP.

Pain-killers

There are three main types of pain-killers commonly used in the medical practice. All these three main types of pain-killers are fairly effective at relieving the pain, though they work better for different kinds of pain. By giving simple pain-killers first to the patients, we could avoid these patients from getting other stronger medication or end up with invasive procedures or surgeries, as what happened to Mr C compared to Captain A in the previous chapters respectively.

They have different side effects and contra-indications, especially to those with kidney diseases. These pain-killers are:

1.   Paracetamol.
2.   Non-Steroidal Anti-Inflammatory Drugs (NSAIDS).
3.   Opioids.

1.   Paracetamol.

Paracetamol is widely used in Malaysia as well as in the UK and Ireland. Even though we have been using paracetamol for a very long time, the exact science of how paracetamol works is still unknown, just like many other things in medicine.

It is believed that it affects the Cyclo-Oxygenase (COX) enzymes in the brain and spinal cord. It can be used to reduce fevers and pain but it does not have the anti-inflammatory properties.

It is also one of the common pain-killers used in the US, but not as common as the Opioids or NSAIDS. In the US, it is commonly known as **acetaminophen,** and you could recognise it by the brand name **Tylenol.**

Paracetamol or Acetaminophen is typically the least strong pain-killer available. Therefore, ***they are generally the safest for use by patients with kidney disease.*** However, overuse or overdose of paracetamol can lead to a liver failure.

2.   <u>**Non-Steroidal Anti-Inflammatory Drugs (NSAIDS).**</u>

Non-Steroidal Anti-Inflammatory Drugs, or NSAIDS, include such common pain-killers as **ibuprofen**, **voltaren**, **synflex**, **ponstan** and **aspirin**. They work by inhibiting the production of cyclo-oxygenase, or COX enzymes. COX enzymes are responsible for the production of prostaglandin, which is what causes inflammation at the site of the wounds in the body.

NSAIDS are *not typically recommended for patients with kidney disease*, with the exception of small doses of aspirin. A low enough dose **to thin the blood and help reduce heart attacks**, has not been shown to be unsafe for kidney patients. Heavy use of high doses of any of the NSAIDs medicine could lead to eventual kidney failure.

3.   <u>**Opioids.**</u>

Opioids refer to the pain-killers that attach themselves to the opioid receptors in the brain and spinal cord, giving a morphine-like pain relief. These actions would give the patients the feeling of sleepiness, euphoria, and anesthetizing effects. These drugs are similar to morphine, which is derived from the opium poppy.

We could also produce opioid drugs using the synthetic opioid derivatives such as the hydrocodone and oxycodone. Opioids are only available in the United States by prescription and are highly regulated because of their addictive side effects. Opioids could also cause damage to the kidneys. Examples of the opioid pain-killers used in Malaysia are ***Tramadol*** and ***Pethidine***.

<u>**The Use of Pain-Killers**</u>

The pain-killer is **one of the most common medicine** that we use in our clinical practice. In the US, they use a lot of Aspirin and other Over the Counter (OTC) pain-killers (e.g. NSAIDS) to treat most of the common complaints such as headaches, fevers, joint pains, body-aches, abdominal pains, toothaches, general feeling of unwell and many more.

In Malaysia we rarely use Aspirin for the above complaints because it is quite a strong medicine. We use a lot of paracetamol instead. That is why paracetamol is allowed to be sold in most shops including the 7-11 stores, restaurants and even in the grocery stores.

If the paracetamol does not work, then we will give other pain-killers, starting with the least strong pain-killers first. By giving the paracetamol and mild pain-killers we could avoid from giving other medicine that is much stronger and with more side effects than these pain-killers.

My late father always complained of back pain, muscle pain or body pain for 10-20 years prior to his death. I needed to give him a constant supply of the paracetamol and voltaren (a mild pain-killer) tablets.

He did not have any kidney problems even though he was having hypertension and taking a lot of paracetamol and mild pain-killers at that time. On a few occasions that I managed to check his blood and urine tests, his kidney function tests, liver function tests and his urine were perfectly normal.

Don't get me wrong here. *I am not saying that taking paracetamol or pain-killer is good.* What I am saying is that if you need to take any medicine for a simple complaint such as a fever, back pain, headaches, body-ache, joint pain, toothache and many other simple complaints then you should take paracetamol or mild pain-killer first.

However, some of the patients refuse to take either the paracetamol or pain killers for simple complaints but request to see a specialist straight away. The problem is if you see a specialist, most of the times you will be given the strongest pain-killers available and a few other strong medicine as well.

Deaths in the USA and UK due to Paracetamol and Other Drugs Overdoses, Suicide, Alcohol and Smoking

Referring to the Table-8 below, in the UK, the number of deaths due to the paracetamol drug poisoning were between 182 to 226 for the years between 2012 to 2017. However, most of these deaths were due to the **intentional** paracetamol overdose.

It meant that most of these people were purposely taking them in much higher doses to commit suicide. Since paracetamol is one of the easiest drugs available over the counter in the UK, they tend to use the paracetamol tablets to commit suicide.

However, there were also some accidental over-dose cases as well, but they were in the minority of cases. It is important to remember that, ***when we use paracetamol at therapeutic levels or normal dosage, it is usually very safe and very effective.***

As comparisons, Table-8 below also shows the number of deaths in the UK due to suicide and deaths related to the alcohol and smoking. Suicide caused between 5,821 to 6,233 deaths between 2012 and 2017. Whereas deaths due to the alcohol and smoking were much higher than the deaths due to the Paracetamol poisoning. Therefore, the numbers of deaths due to the Paracetamol poisoning was very low if compared to deaths due to other form of suicides, alcohol or smoking.

SER	YEAR	CAUSE OF DEATH							
		Drug Poisoning US	PCM Poisoning UK	SUICIDE		ALCOHOL		SMOKING	
				US	UK	US	UK	US	UK
1.	2012	41,502	182	40,600	5,981	about 88,000 /year	8,367	about 480,000 /year	79,900
2.	2013	43,982	226	41,149	6,233		8,416		79,700
3.	2014	47,055	200	42,773	6,122		8,697		80,000
4.	2015	52,372	197	44,193	6,188		8,758		79,100
5.	2016	63,632	219	44,695	5,965		7,327		77,900
6.	2017	72,306	218	47,173	5,821		-		-
7.	2018	-	-	48,344	-		-		-

Table-8: Number of deaths due to paracetamol poisoning, suicide, death-related to alcohol and smoking. Sources: CDC, US and NHS, UK.
Notes:
1.   Alcohol-related death include Alcoholic liver disease, Alcohol-induced acute and chronic pancreatitis, Alcoholic cardiomyopathy, Alcoholic myopathy, Excess alcohol blood levels, Accidental poisoning by and exposure to alcohol, Intentional self-poisoning by and exposure to alcohol etc.
2.   Smoking-related death include deaths due to increase risks to coronary artery disease, stroke, lung cancer, chronic obstructive lung disease etc.

In other words, ***smoking and drinking alcohol are much more dangerous than taking the paracetamol.*** In the UK in 2016, alcohol-related deaths caused 33 times or 3,300% more deaths than the paracetamol poisoning. Whereas smoking caused 355 times or 35,500% more deaths than the paracetamol poisoning. This means that death due to paracetamol overdose is very small. Most of these overdoses were due to people who wanted to commit suicide anyway. But many people don't give a second thought about how dangerous the alcohol and smoking are, but very worried about the side effects of the paracetamol tablets.

In the US, deaths due to drug poisoning or drug overdoses are much higher than the UK. Since they are not using as much paracetamol as the UK and Malaysia do, drug overdoses in the US are due to other drugs. The most common drugs involved are the opioids, most commonly the heroin.

There are a few things that you can do to ensure that you are taking the pain-killers properly:

1.   Always consult your doctors before using a pain-killer.

2.   Follow package directions on the OTC pain-killers. Don't take continuously for more than 10 days and consult your doctor if the pain continues.

3.   Avoid pain-killers that include mixed analgesics such as ibuprofen, caffeine and acetaminophen. The mixed pain-killers are more likely to cause side effects *for kidney patients*.

4.   Don't take pain-killers with alcohol.

Low Blood Pressure in Women– It's not a cause of dizzy spells or fainting attacks and it is not a Medical Problem

Some people believe that a low blood pressure causes the dizziness or fainting attack. I had many patients especially the women that came to the clinics to check for their Blood Pressures because they thought that they had low BP problems. Most of them would have other complaints as well such as the headaches, migraines or vertigo.

These are not true. There are many people that have low BPs but never complain of any problems. And many people that complain of having dizzy spells, giddiness or fainting attacks have normal BPs.

During my services in the military, I had the privilege of doing medical check-ups for a lot of normal people. These people included the military personnel (there were about 120,000 of military personnel at any time, most of them had to do the routine medical check-ups once for every 4 years, some needed to do it once for every 2 years and some of them needed to do it every year depending on their age, rank, type of job etc. Now most of them need to do it every 2 years instead of every 4 years), military reserve personnel which was about 300,000 men and women, people that wanted to join the military either as the recruits or cadets, students that wanted to go for the PLKN training and many more.

In short, every year we did thousands of medical check-ups for normal people. We found out that about 50% of the women and 10% of the men would have low Blood Pressures. Some of these women would have very low BPs of 80/50, or 70/40 and we even found some of them that had BPs of 50/30 or 40/30. However, none of these women complained of any dizzy spells, giddiness or fainting attacks. In fact, all of these women could run 5 or 10 kms without any problems.

These young women were at the beginning of their careers in the military. Therefore, they would have many military training, tests or exercises that they had to do and pass. If they did not do all of these training, tests and exercises then their military careers would become a problem. Somehow they never thought of complaining of having not only for the dizzy spells, giddiness or fainting attacks, but also for other complains such as the headaches, migraines or vertigo, regardless of their blood pressure readings.

I also used to work at one of the military hospitals for 3 years and at another training center for another 2 years. Both of these places had many young recruits or officers doing their military training. As far as I could remember, nobody died, or developed any form of complications or just collapsed during their training due to the low

BPs. We would have known about it because it would become a major issue in the military.

Even when I was looking after the Medical Out-Patient Department (MOPD) at one of the military hospitals, we did not have any patients with a low blood pressure. I am sure that if there were doctors that would refer any patient to this MOPD for a low BP, not only would my consultant be screaming mad, I would do the same for unnecessary referrals.

For women, the lower the BPs that they have is the better. The reason is that their BPs are made that way to prepare for the increase in their BPs when they get pregnant. Most women would have their BPs increased due to the pregnancy, especially after 28 weeks of pregnancy.

If their BPs are at 80/50, even if they are increased by 50/30 during pregnancy it would still be normal at 130/80. If their BPs are already at 120/70, which most people regard as not low BPs, then if their BPs are increased by the same rate of 50/30 they would have very high BPs at 170/100. This high BP of 170/100 during pregnancy is very dangerous and could kill both the mother and the baby.

The problem is that some doctors want to give a reason for these women's complaints of frequent dizzy spells, giddiness or fainting attacks. So they blame the low BPs that cause the symptoms.

Even a patient that fainted for more than 8 hours as in the Case No. 20 above did not have a low BP. Then all these problems of dizzy spells, giddiness or fainting attacks are all in the minds, i.e in those who are thinking that they are having all of these problems because of their low BPs.

CHAPTER 8

THE COMMON COMPLAINT AND TREATMENT

C.   UPPER RESPIRATORY TRACT INFECTIONS (URTIs)
- Common Cold and Flu

'Common Cold: An ailment cured in two weeks with a doctor's care and in fourteen days without it'.

-    *Anonymous*

The Upper Respiratory Tract Infections or URTIs are the most common complaints seen at the General Practitioner's (GP's) Clinics in Malaysia. In general, they are mild illnesses, easy to treat and most patients would fully recover from the infections without any further complications.

However, this topic is the most difficult one for me to write. I hope that I do not give the wrong information to the readers from what I intended to do.

A lot of people in Malaysia are really scared of this infection. Many of the patients are regularly asking me to refer them to the hospitals even though their symptoms are very mild. These hospital appointments or admissions are mostly **unnecessary**.

They just need a simple treatment with simple medication. They need to drink plenty of fluids and rest at home. The treatment given is directed at managing the symptoms while our bodies' own immune system fights the infection.

Antibiotics are of no use against the URTI viruses and should not be used unless there is a bacterial infection. They do not need to take the anti-viral medicine either unless they are in the high risk groups.

Case No. 28

Parent A,

2018, England, UK.

My wife and I went to England in 2018 to attend our daughter's graduation ceremony at her university. There were a few other parents attending the same event. One of the parents suddenly fell sick with a fever and a few other symptoms such as the runny nose, coughs, a sore-throat and a body-ache.

He was one of the high ranking officer in the company that he was working with, and had many medical benefits from that company. He was used to being admitted to the private hospitals in Malaysia for similar complaints.

Unfortunately there were no private hospitals at where we were staying. Even to see the general practitioner there would take a few days just to get the appointment. It was almost impossible for him to be referred to the NHS hospital urgently.

So he decided to go back to Malaysia as early as possible to get himself admitted to the hospital. He contacted his airline and requested to change his return ticket to Kuala Lumpur on the earliest possible date available. He was asked to go to London and wait for the airline to get the new ticket sorted out.

Since it was a summer, it took the airline a few days to get the earlier flight confirmed, which was only 1 or 2 days earlier than the flight that he was originally supposed to take. Because of this flight changes, he had to pay quite a lot of money for the new ticket and for the accommodation in London. He also had to cancel all the travels that he had planned to do with his family in the UK.

Whereas if I were to have similar problems, I would just take plenty of paracetamol tablets, and may be a cough syrup and anti-histamine tablets for the cough and the flu, which I can buy either at the supermarkets or pharmacies there, re-hydrate myself with plenty of iced water, and continue with the travel plans.

Even in the UK and US, their treatment for the URTI infections are almost the same as I mentioned above, even though they have a very high number of deaths among their URTI's patient.

<u>**Acute Upper Respiratory Tract Infections (URTIs)**</u>

The respiratory tract is divided into two different types based on its anatomy, as described below:

1. <u>**The Upper Respiratory Tract**</u>:
    a.   It includes the mouth, nose, sinus, throat, larynx (voice box) and trachea (windpipe).
    b.   ***Upper respiratory tract infections are divided into two main groups, either the Common Colds or the Flu Infections.***

2. <u>**The Lower Respiratory Tract**</u>:
    a.   It includes the bronchial tubes and the lungs.
    b.   Bronchitis, bronchiolitis in children and pneumonia (lung infections) are infections of the lower respiratory tract.

The Acute Upper Respiratory Tract Infections or Acute URTIs are the most common complaints of the respiratory tract infections as I mentioned above. Every year we could easily have millions of people in Malaysia who are infected with the URTIs.

The acute URTIs are divided into 2 different major illnesses, *the Common Colds and the Flu infections.* Even though both of them have similar symptoms and signs but they are classified as 2 different infections.

(1)   <u>Common Cold</u>

The Common Cold is more common than the Flu infection in Malaysia and in other tropical countries, whereas the Flu is more common in the temperate and cold countries. In general, the Common Cold is the mild form of the acute URTIs.

They usually cause mild signs and symptoms of the viral infections. They will not cause any deaths. More than 200 different viruses can cause the Common Cold infections. Examples of these viruses are:

1.   Rhinovirus - responsible for at least 60% of the Common Cold infections.

2.   Corona Virus.

3.   Respiratory Syncytial Virus (RSV).

4.   Para-influenza virus.

5.   Adenovirus.

People "catch" colds when they are exposed to the airborne viruses. Usually the virus spreads from person to person in the respiratory droplets from sneezing or coughing. Most resolve within a week or 2 weeks. If symptoms persist after more than 2 weeks, then it may be an indication to seek medical evaluations.

In the Common Cold, the patients usually would present the following symptoms:

1.   Mild fever.

2.   Nasal symptoms i.e sneezing, nasal discharge, nasal congestion, runny nose.

3.   Sore throat.

4.   Coughs.

5.   Headaches.

6.   bodyache or joint pain.

7.   Rashes.

Most people with the Common Cold infections can be diagnosed by their signs and symptoms. Therefore, you do not need to have any blood or urine tests, or chest x-ray done. There is no cure for the Common Cold.

As mentioned above and I repeat here: Antibiotics are of no use against the Common Cold viruses and should not be used unless there is a bacterial infection. Again, The treatment given is just to make ourselves feel better while our bodies' own immune system fights the infection.

(2)   **Influenza or Flu Infection**

Since Influenza viruses can cause the severe form of the upper respiratory tract infections, it is classified as a different illness. It is usually called the *Influenza infection*, or the *Seasonal Flu* or just *the Flu*. The word *Flu* is derived from part of the word **Influenza.**

The Flu is more common in the temperate and cold countries as the virus is more active at low temperature. I will explain in more details about Influenza viruses below because many people in Malaysia are really worried about them.

Influenza Virus

In general, the Flu infection is worse than the Common Cold infection, and the symptoms are more common and intense. Comparison between the symptoms of the Influenza and the Common Cold infections are as in Table-9 below:

SER	SIGNS & SYMPTOMS	INFLUENZA (FLU)	COMMON COLD
1.	Symptoms and onset	Abrupt	Gradual
2.	Fever	Temp. >37.8° C, lasting 3-4 days	Temp. <37.8°C.
3.	Cough	Common, Sometimes severe	Mild to Moderate
4.	Aches	Usual	Slight
5.	Chills	Fairly Common	Uncommon
6.	Fatigue, Weakness	Usual	Sometimes
7.	Sneezing	Sometimes	Common
8.	Stuffy Nose	Sometimes	Common
9.	Sore throat	Sometimes	Common
10.	Chest Discomfort	Common	Mild to Moderate
11.	Headache	Common	Rare

Table-9: Comparison between the symptoms of the Influenza and the Common Cold infections.
(Source:https://www.healthpartners.com/blog/cold-vs-flu-how-to-spot-the-symptoms/)

The name Seasonal Flu is actually misleading because you can get the flu at any time of the year. The viruses are transmitted throughout the populations all year round but you are **more likely to get it in winter.**

There are a few reasons why the flu is much more common in the winter:

1.   In one study done using guinea pigs, they found that by varying air temperature and humidity in the guinea pigs' quarters, they

discovered that the flu transmission between the guinea pigs was maximum at 41°F (5°C -winter temperature). It declined as the temperature rose until, by 86°F (30°C -summer temperature) the viruses were not transmitted at all. Therefore, the flu transmission is best in winter and could stop in summer. *(Source: Influenza Virus Transmission Is Dependent on Relative Humidity and Temperature.-Anice C Lowen, Samira Mubareka, John Steel, Peter Palese. Published: October 19, 2007. Website:https://doi.org/10.1371/journal.ppat.0030151)*

2.	The Flu viruses spread through the air, unlike the Common Cold viruses, which primarily spread by direct contact when people touch surfaces that have been touched by someone with a cold or shake hands with someone who is infected with the virus. Flu viruses are more stable in cold air (winter), and low humidity helps the virus particles remain in the air. Since the flu viruses float in the air in little respiratory droplets, when the air is humid (summer), those droplets pick up water, grow larger and fall to the ground.

3.	During winter, people are usually indoors and children are at school. They are crowded together and this makes it much easier to pass the flu to the other person.

4.	Cold temperatures lead to drier air, which may dehydrate our mucous membranes, preventing the body from effectively defending against the flu or the Common Cold virus infections.

There are three different types of Influenza viruses: The Influenza Types A, B, and C.

1.	**Influenza Type A virus or Type A Flu virus**. Type A Flu virus is capable of infecting birds and some mammals such as humans, pigs and horses.

2.	**Influenza Type B virus or Type B Flu virus**. Unlike Type A Flu virus, Type B Flu virus is found only in humans. Type B Flu virus may cause **a less severe reaction** than Type A Flu virus, but occasionally Type B Flu virus can still be extremely harmful.

3.	**Influenza Type C virus or Type C Flu virus**. Type C Flu virus infection generally cause a mild respiratory illness and are not thought to cause epidemics.

Human Influenza A and B viruses cause seasonal flu epidemics almost every winter in the Western World. Type A Flu virus is constantly changing or mutating and is generally responsible for the large flu epidemics.

A small change to the genetic makeup of influenza strains is referred to as ***antigenic drift***, while a major change is called ***antigenic shift***. While these designations are mainly relevant to the scientists, they help explain why you can contract the flu more than once and why the influenza vaccine is changed annually.

These changes i.e the antigenic drift and antigenic shift are the reasons why only the epidemic Influenza A virus that can sometimes become **pandemic** i.e. an epidemic of an influenza A virus that spreads on a worldwide scale and infects a large proportion of the world population. (Basically a pandemic is much larger than an epidemic). They become a pandemic with the emergence of a new and very different sub-type or strain of the Influenza A virus.

Influenza B viruses are not classified by subtype, but can be further broken down into lineages and strains. Currently circulating influenza B viruses belong to one of two lineages: B/Yamagata and B/Victoria. *Influenza B does not cause pandemic.*

1.   <u>Influenza A Virus</u>

As I mentioned above, Influenza A virus or Type A Flu Virus is the most dangerous among the different types of Influenza viruses. Type A flu virus is constantly changing and is generally responsible for the large flu epidemics which can spread all over the world to become a pandemic attack.

The Influenza A viruses are further divided into **different sub-types** based on **two proteins found on the surface of the virus**: the **Hemagglutinin (H)** and the **Neuraminidase (N)**. Many people are familiar with this H and N subtype for example the *Influenza A H1N1*. There are 18 different Hemagglutinin sub-types and 11 different Neuraminidase sub-types. (H1 to H18 and N1 to N11 respectively).

Therefore, we could have an Influenza A subtype H1N1, H1N2 until H1N11, then we would have the subtype H2N1, H2N2 until

H2N11 and so on until we have the subtype H18N11. All together, we have almost 200 different sub-types of Influenza A. Current sub-types of influenza A viruses found in people are **Influenza A H1N1** and **Influenza A H3N2** viruses. *The Influenza A H1N1 is best known for causing widespread outbreaks, including the epidemics and pandemics.*

There is no other dangerous threat of infectious disease in the world as the threat of an influenza epidemic or pandemic. Well, now we also have a pandemic from a **corona virus infection.** We have had four past influenza pandemics that affect the whole world, **but more in the temperate and cold countries.**

1.   <u>**The 1918 Pandemic (H1N1)- Spanish Flu.**</u>

(Source: Google- Centers for Disease Control and Prevention- Pandemic Flu. https://www.cdc.gov/flu/pandemic-resources/1918-pandemic-h1n1.html)

a.   The 1918 influenza pandemic was the most severe pandemic in recent history. It was caused by an Influenza A (H1N1) virus with genes of avian (bird) origin. Although there is no universal consensus regarding where the virus originated, it spread worldwide during 1918-1919.

b.   In the United States, it was first identified in a military personnel in the Spring 1918. It was estimated that about 500 million people or one-third of the world's population became infected with this virus. The number of deaths was estimated to be at least 50 million worldwide with about 675,000 occurring in the United States.

c.   Mortality was high in people younger than 5 years old, 20-40 years old, and 65 years and older. The high mortality in healthy people, including those in the 20-40 year age group, was a unique feature of this pandemic.

2.   <u>**The 1957-1958 Pandemic (H2N2 virus)- Asian Flu.**</u>

(Source:https://www.cdc.gov/flu/pandemic-resources/19571958pandemic. html).

In February 1957, a new Influenza A (H2N2) virus emerged in East Asia, triggering a pandemic ("Asian Flu"). It was first reported in Singapore in February 1957, Hong Kong in April 1957, and in the

United States in the Summer 1957. The estimated number of deaths was 1.1 million worldwide and 116,000 in the United States.

3.   <u>The 1968 pandemic (H3N2)- Hong Kong Flu.</u>

(Source:https://www.cdc.gov/flu/pandemic-resources/1968-pandemic.html)

a.   It was caused by an Influenza A (H3N2) virus comprised of two genes from an avian Influenza A virus. It was first noted in the United States in September 1968.

b.   The estimated number of deaths was 1 million world-wide and about 100,000 in the United States. Most deaths were in people 65 years and older. The Influenza A (H3N2) virus continues to circulate worldwide today as a seasonal Influenza A virus.

4.   <u>The 2009 pandemic (a novel H1N1)- H1N1/09 Flu.</u>

(Source:https://www.cdc.gov/flu/pandemic-resources/2009-h1n1-pandemic. html)

a.   In the spring of 2009, a novel (new) Influenza A H1N1 virus emerged. It was detected first in the United States and spread quickly across the United States and the world. This new Influenza A H1N1 virus contained a unique combination of influenza genes not previously identified in animals or people.

b.   This virus was designated as an Influenza A H1N1/09 virus. Few young people had any existing immunity (as detected by antibody response) to the Influenza A H1N1/09 virus, but nearly one-third of people over the age of 60 had antibodies against this virus, most likely from an exposure to an older Influenza A (H1N1) virus earlier in their lives.

c.   The CDC, US estimated that there were 60.8 million cases, 274,304 hospitalizations, and 12,469 deaths in the United States due to the H1N1/09 virus. The CDC also estimated that between 151,700 and 575,400 people worldwide died from the 2009 H1N1 virus infection during the first year the virus circulated.

For most people, the Flu only causes a few days of feeling sick with symptoms of fever, coughs, runny nose, sore throat, chills, bodyaches or rashes. However, for certain groups of the populations, the Flu can be more dangerous and can become life threatening infections. These vulnerable groups of people are:

1.	Children under the age of five, especially those two years and younger.

2.	Adults over 65 years of age.

3.	Pregnant women.

4.	People with serious medical conditions such as the chronic lung diseases, diabetes, asthma, heart diseases, cancer, kidney disorders, or blood disorders.

5.	Individuals on immuno-suppressive agents (e.g. HIV, patient on chemotherapy).

6.	Morbidly obese people.

The single best way to prevent a seasonal flu infection and to have the less severe form of the infection according to WHO is to get vaccinated each year. Good health habits like covering your cough and washing your hands often can help stop the spread of the germs and prevent other respiratory illnesses. WHO currently recommends annual influenza vaccinations for the following people (especially if you live in the temperate and cold countries):

1.	Pregnant women.

2.	Children between the ages of 6 months and 5 years.

3.	Elderly people above 65.

4.	People suffering from the chronic medical conditions.

5.	Health care workers.

THE BURDEN OF THE COMMON COLD AND FLU INFECTIONS

### 1.	Common Cold

As I mentioned above, the majority of people infected with the common cold infections are suffering from the mild symptoms of the URTIs such as a mild fever or no fever at all, slight coughs, a mild sore throat or mild nasal complaints. Most resolve within a week or 2 weeks with simple medication and rehydration without any further complications.

In the tropical countries, the common cold infections almost never cause any deaths, and even the flu infections rarely cause any deaths either, except during the pandemic infection.

2.   <u>Influenza</u>

In contrast, the Influenza infections can cause a lot of deaths especially in the temperate and cold countries. In general, the Flu infections cause more severe form of illnesses and could lead to death more than the Common Cold infections. The Flu infections can also cause the pandemic infections where they spread quickly across countries or continents around the world and affect millions of people.

Unfortunately, we do not have accurate statistic datas on the number of acute URTI cases in Malaysia. For example if I want to find out how many people in Malaysia suffer from the URTIs, from the Common Colds or from the Influenza infections every year, I could not find a reliable website like the Centers for Disease Control and Prevention (CDC) in the US or the Public Health England in the UK. Most of the time the data available from different websites were contradicting with each other.

The reason for the absence of our statistics for the URTIs, either the Common Colds or the Flu Infections in Malaysia could be due to the following points:

1.   Malaysian Doctors do not have to report the URTI cases to the health authorities because they are not dangerous infections.

2.   The government hospitals and clinics, and most GP clinics rarely test for the Common Cold or Influenza viruses on their patients.

3.   Since we do not have to report these cases to the health authorities and we rarely test for the Common Cold or Influenza viruses, therefore there are no proper records or statistics about them available.

Some of the websites, especially the ones from overseas would put the Influenza and Pneumonia (inflammation of the lungs i.e.

serious lung infections) as one of the leading cause of deaths in Malaysia. This is not true. In my 25 years' experience as a doctor, Influenza infections rarely cause any deaths in Malaysia, except during the Pandemic Influenza A/H1N1 in 2009. Even during that time, the number of deaths were less than 100.

Since in the temperate and cold countries Influenza is a common cause of pneumonia, and sometimes they cannot prove that it is the Influenza virus that causes the pneumonia, therefore *they combine both Influenza and Pneumonia as one of the leading causes of death*. But most cases of the influenza infections never lead to pneumonia, especially in the tropical countries like Malaysia. But those that do, they tend to be more severe and deadly.

In the US, the CDC estimates that every year Influenza has resulted in between 23.5 million to 45 million illnesses (the number of people infected with the virus will be much higher since most patients won't have any symptoms), between 140,000 to 810,000 hospitalisations and between 22,000 to 61,000 deaths annually since 2012. *(Source: Disease Burden of Influenza - CDC).*

They also estimate that the Flu infections cost to the US about $87 billion per year. This figure is better shown in Table-10 below.

SER	COST OF FLU INFECTION TO USA EVERY YEAR	
1.	No. of People Infected	23.5 million to 45.5 million people
2.	Hospitalisation	140,000 to 810,000 patients
3.	Cost in US$	$87 billion dollars
4.	Deaths	22,000 - 61,000

Table-10: Cost of The Flu Infection to the US.
(Source:Google- 'Healthline- The Flu: Facts, Statistics, and You'.
https://www.healthline.com/health/influenza/facts-and-statistics#Costs)

a.   <u>**Number of Deaths due to the Flu Infections in the USA, England and Malaysia**</u>

In the temperate and cold countries, the Influenza infections can cause a lot of deaths. In the US for example, there were more than 22,000 deaths in every winter season since 2012/2013, as shown in Table-11 below. During 2017/2018 winter, the U.S. government estimates that 61,099 Americans died of the flu, the disease's highest death toll in at least four decades.

(Source: https://edition. cnn. com/2018/09/26/health/flu-deaths-2017--2018-cdc-bn/index. html)

SER	SEASON	NO. OF DEATH		
		US	ENGLAND	MALAYSIA
1.	2012-2013	42,570	-	?0
2.	2013-2014	37,930	3,107	?0
3.	2014-2015	51,376	28,330	?0
4.	2015-2016	22,705	11,875	?0
5.	2016-2017	38,230	18,009	?0
6.	2017-2018	61,099	26,408	?1
7.	2018-2019	34,157	3,966	?0
8.	2019-2020	43,000 *est*	7,990	?0

Table-11: Number of Deaths Due to Influenza infection in US, England and Malaysia.

Source: 1. cdc.gov/flu/about/burden/2018-2019 (according to the year).html
2.Public Health England. Surveillance of influenza and other respiratory viruses in the UK. (Winter 2018-2019-Page 51, Table 7)

In England the number of deaths were between 3,107 to 34,300 for the same period of time. This fluctuation of number of deaths was due to the virulence (the severity or harmfulness of the virus infection) of the flu virus in that particular year. Whereas In Malaysia I could not find any report of deaths directly due to an influenza infection except there was one case in 2017.

Influenza and Pneumonia

Influenza and Pneumonia is an important cause of mortality in the temperate and cold countries, especially in the winter. Pneumonia is a serious lung infection or inflammation of the lungs. Since Influenza is a common cause of pneumonia, and sometimes they cannot prove that it is the Influenza virus that causes the pneumonia, therefore ***they combine both Influenza and Pneumonia as one of the leading causes of death.***

Most cases of the flu never lead to pneumonia, but those that do, tend to be more severe and deadly. Pneumonia that is caused by

Influenza virus are usually common among younger children, the elderly, pregnant women, or those with certain chronic health conditions.

Therefore, Influenza & Pneumonia infection is a very big and serious medical problems in the temperate and cold countries. In the US, Influenza and Pneumonia is the eighth leading cause of deaths. As Table-12 shows below, they cause more than 50,000 deaths every year since 2012.

SER	NO. OF DEATHS DUE TO INFLUENZA & PNEUMONIA IN US	
	Year	No. of Deaths
1.	2012	50,636
2.	2013	56,979
3.	2014	55,227
4.	2015	57,063
5.	2016	51,537
6.	2017	55,672

Table-12: Number of Deaths Due to Influenza and Pneumonia in the US.
(Source: CDC: National Vital Statistics. Death: Final Data for 2017(according to year). Website:https://www.cdc.gov/nchs/data/nvsr/nvsr68/nvsr68_09-508.pdf 2.)

There are more deaths due to Influenza and Pneumonia in the winter because of a few reasons:

1. The Flu infections which cause the pneumonia are more common in the winter as mentioned above.

2. There are always more deaths in the winter for any reasons than any other seasons, particularly among elderly people. Since there are much higher cases of Flu infections in the winter and the colder weather increases other respiratory problems, therefore there are more deaths in the winter due to the Flu infections as well.

3. Cold weather stresses the heart and the lungs as the body works to maintain its core temperature. In vulnerable patients like patients with heart problems, diabetes, chronic lung diseases, elderly people or those with cancer, a flu infection can easily kill the patient whose body is already under stress due to the cold weather.

1. <u>Treatment of the Flu infections in the USA</u>

SER	SEASON	ESTIMATES OF INFLUENZA DISEASE BURDEN- UNITED STATES OF AMERICA			
		Patients with Symptoms	*Medical Visits*	*Hospitalisation*	*No. Of Death*
1	2018-19	35,520,883 (100%)	16,520,350 (46.5%)	490,561 (1.38%)	34,157 (0.10%)
2	2017-18	44,802,629 (100%)	20,731,323 (46.3%)	808,129 (1.80%)	61,099 (0.14%)
3	2016-17	29,220,523 (100%)	13,633,446 (46.7%)	496,912 (1.70%)	38,230 (0.13%)
4	2015-16	23,504,319 (100%)	10,642,006 (45.3%)	276,198 (1.18%)	22,705 (0.10%)
5	2014-15	30,165,452 (100%)	14,407,876 (47.8%)	590,869 (1.96%)	51,376 (0.17%)
6	2013-14	29,739,994 (100%)	13,192,531 (44.4%)	346,912 (1.17%)	37,930 (0.13%)
7	2012-13	33,679,171 (100%)	15,799,206 (46.9%)	571,382 (1.70%)	42,570 (0.13%)

Table-13: Estimates of The Influenza Disease Burden in The US.
Source: cdc.gov/flu/about/burden/2018-2019 (according to the year).html

Table-13 above shows that for ***the majority of patients with the Flu infections in the US from 2012 to 2019 were not admitted to the hospitals***. Out of 23.5 to 44.5 million infected people that were down with the symptoms of the flu infections, only between 276,198 to 808,129 patients that were admitted to the hospitals. In other words, only between 1.18% to 1.8% of the infected patients with the illnesses were admitted to the hospitals in the US between 2012-2019.

Even with more than **22,000 deaths every year** due to the Influenza infections since 2012, **the majority of patients in the US were advised to rest at home**. Most of the patients did not even go and see their doctors at all. Less than 50% of the cases went to see their doctors and less than 2% of the cases were admitted to the hospitals.

The Flu treatment in the US is very simple and straightforward. Their Centers for Disease Control and Prevention department has produced a guideline's booklet for the flu patients and their carers to follow, the latest was published in December 2010.

(Refer: 'The Flu: Caring for someone at home' booklet published in Dec 2010).

They advice the people that are infected with the Flu infections to follow these 5 steps *(Refer to Page 2 of the booklet)*:

1.	Stay at home and rest.

2.	Avoid close contact with healthy people in your house so you won't make them sick.

3.	Drink plenty of water and other clear fluids to prevent fluid loss (dehydration).

4.	Treat fever and cough with medicine that you can buy at the store.

5.	If you get very sick or are pregnant or have a medical condition that put you in higher risks of flu complications such as asthma, call your doctor. You **might need** (not mandatory) anti-viral medicine to treat the flu.

I think the guidelines are very clear. If you think that you are infected with the Flu infection (including the Influenza A H1N1 or H3N2), you don't have to go to the hospitals straight away.

Stay at home first. Don't mix with other healthy people, drink plenty of fluids and take simple medicine (Over The Counters-OTC) that you can buy from the supermarkets or pharmacies. Only at risk patients that need to see their doctors, and majority of them do not need to be admitted to the hospitals.

They also give the following advises in the same booklet:

1.	Keep cooler or pitcher with ice and drinks.

2.	Take ice chips or frozen ice pops to numb the throat and get fluids into the body.

3.	Take Acetaminophen (Paracetamols) or ibuprofen for the pain.

There are 2 interesting advises that the CDC gave above, to take cold water or drinks, and to suck the ice pops or ice cubes for the sore-throat. Even though the flu infections in the US usually take place in the cold winter, but they advice the patients to take a cold water instead of a hot water.

These 2 advises look simple, but I think they explain the reasons why so many of the Malaysian patients take a much longer time to recover from a simple common cold or a flu infection. Sometimes they do not recover even after 3 or 4 weeks of taking 2 or 3 different antibiotics and an anti-viral medicine at the same time.

In Malaysia, most of the patients that are infected with the common colds or the flu infections would specifically take warm or hot water throughout their illnesses. They also take the hot soups as well. At the same time they prefer not to take any paracetamol tablets because they think that the paracetamol is a very dangerous medicine.

But they have no problems in taking the antibiotics or anti-viral medicine. Drinking warm or hot water will keep their body temperatures higher and they would increase the inflammation in their throats. Whereas we need to reduce the temperatures and reduce the inflammation in our throats to treat these infections.

They also advice that only a minority of the patients i.e the patients in the high risk groups such as the patients with Asthma, Diabetes, Chronic Obstructive Airways Disease (COAD), Heart problems or Pregnant ladies that may require the anti-viral medicine.

2. <u>Treatment of the Flu infections in the UK</u>

The treatment for the URTI infections in the UK are almost the same as the treatment given in the US and at the government hospitals in Malaysia. One day my nephew who was studying in the UK fell sick with a fever, coughs, a sore throat and a runny nose. He went to see his GP, but could not see him on that day. He was given an appointment in 4 days time.

He immediately messaged me through the phone for a consultation. I advised him to buy a few medicine at the supermarket and rest at home. In the UK, if you are sick with the signs and symptoms of an Influenza infection, you don't even have to get the Medical Certificates (MCs) from the doctors if you are not fit to go to work for the first 7 days of the year. You can just use a self-certification saying that you are not fit for work on that day.

They also advice their patients to take any of the Over The Counter (OTC) medicine that they could buy from the supermarkets or from the pharmacies. They have a very good section in almost all of their supermarkets that sell a good selection of the OTC medicine. You only need to see the doctor for the MCs from the 8th day onwards. Now their General Practitioner's association wants these 7 days of self-certification to be increased to 14 days for each year.

Yes, in the UK, their General Practitioners are saying that if you are really sick and unable to go to work, you don't have to go and see them. You just take whatever medicine you have at home or whatever medicine you can buy over the counter from the supermarkets or pharmacies, and just inform your employer that you are sick.

They don't even ask them to come for a check-up. Why? Because they knew that most of these problems were simple cases that did not require any special treatment. They would recover with just the simple medicine that they could buy over the counters in most supermarkets or pharmacies.

3. Treatment of the Flu and Common Cold infections in Malaysia

However, it is very different in Malaysia. Most patients would ask the doctors to really check their bodies for any sign of infections. They expect their doctors to check their temperatures, lungs, abdomens and their throats even though they do not have sore throats. They also want the blood tests to be done, and sometimes request to be referred to the hospitals urgently.

Although in theory, it is a good practice to detect any dangerous infections early. However, in the best practice in medicine, for many cases like these, it is a bad idea to ask your doctors to simply check your whole bodies and to refer you to the hospitals, as what happened to the Girl A in Case No. 11 above, who died in the ICU at the hospital from a simple Common Cold Infection.

As Malaysia enjoys a tropical weather year round with temperatures ranging from a mild 20°C to a hot 30°C average throughout the year, even the Influenza infection is not a big issue as in the temperate and cold countries. Death due to the Common Colds or Flu Infections are very rare in Malaysia, except during the Pandemic Influenza A (H1N1) in 2009. That is why the government hospitals rarely do blood tests to check for the Influenza infections at their clinics or hospitals.

Since most of the common colds and flu infections in Malaysia recover fully without any complications, the government hospitals prefer to treat both infections symptomatically with simple medication. They rarely admit the patients to the ward. The government hospitals usually do not want to admit all these patients unless they are in the high risk groups.

As mentioned above, both infections of the Common Cold and the Flu in Malaysia only cause minor illnesses, therefore, their treatment are almost the same. The treatment is directed at relieving the signs and symptoms of the infections, which include:

1.	Anti-Pyretic (to reduce fever) and pain relievers for the fever, a sore throat and headaches. The most commonly used anti-pyretic and pain relievers in Malaysia is a Paracetamol tablet.

2.	Anti-histamine tablets or decongestant nasal sprays for the nasal symptoms.

3.	Cough syrups.

4.	Drink plenty of fluids. For me, cold plain water is the best, as advised by the CDC, US. For older kids or adult patients you could also take any one of the isotonic drinks such as the 100 Plus or Revive.

5.	Avoid caffeine and alcohol, which can dehydrate you.

6.   Relieve your sore throat. Take any lozenges, saltwater gargles, any ready-made gargles or you could take ice cubes or ice cream to numb the throat and reduce the inflammation.

7.   Rest. If possible, stay home from work or school especially if you have a high fever or a bad cough or are drowsy after taking the medication. This will give you a chance to rest as well as reduce the chances that you will infect other people.

They rarely give antibiotics to the patients, because both of the infections are due to viruses, which do not respond to the antibiotics. They also rarely give the anti-viral medicine, unless the patients are in the high risk groups and really need them. In fact, we never gave any anti-viral medicine to our common cold and flu patients during my time working in the military service.

Unfortunately, I have many patients at the private sectors that are taking not only the antibiotics, but also taking the anti-viral medicine at the same time. They also insist on either doing the blood tests or throat swabs to check for the Flu virus or to be referred to the hospitals. Most of the time they would be immediately admitted to the hospitals if their Flu tests are positive.

Even in England and the US, where they have thousands of people die due to the Flu infections every year, they rarely admit their patients. Case No. 21 below shows that even in these extreme cases the government hospitals still did not want to admit these patients.

Case No. 29
Multiple Army Personnel,
Malaysian Border Patrols.

I was a medical officer at one of the air-force bases in North Malaysia when our clinic received an urgent call. They told us to be ready to receive about 10 sick army personnel. They would be brought out from the jungle with a helicopter and they would land on a field nearby our clinic. These were our soldiers that were protecting our borders with Thailand to prevent anybody from entering the country illegally.

Apparently, they had been having high fevers in the jungle for a few days and one of their colleague had died. When the helicopter landed, they were immediately brought to our clinic. When I checked, almost everybody was still having the fevers. Some of them also complained of severe headaches, body pain, joint pain, and feeling lethargic. More than half of them had high temperatures of above 38°C.

I gave a few days of rest for the soldiers that had temperatures below 38°C. The soldiers that had high temperatures of above 38°C were referred to the General Hospital near-by. However, about one or two hours later I was told that all of them were asked to go back and rest at home.

I assumed that the hospital did not even do a simple blood test for these soldiers because of the quick decision to send them home. Fortunately, all these army personnel recovered from their infections without any complications.

<u>Sore-throats</u>

A sore throat is one of the simple symptoms that the patients complaint, either alone or with other symptoms like a fever, coughs, or a runny nose. Initially I did not even notice about this problem. I always thought that it was a simple complaint. Whenever my family and I suffer from the sore throats, we would always take the paracetamol tablets for the fever and pain, and plenty of cold water or iced water to cool down the throat and to reduce the throat inflammation.

As long as the fever is not persistently high (>38°C) for a few days and you could still drink water, then you just need to take the paracetamol tablets (even without the fever) to reduce the pain and take plenty of cold water, or iced water or even ice cream to reduce the throat inflammations as mentioned above. For the ice cream, it does not matter what flavour it is, as long as it is cold. It is nothing to do with the **vanilla flavour** as believed by many Malaysians. The best ice cream is the Malaysian homemade ice cream because it mostly contains ice.

Therefore, rarely my grandparents, my parents, my wife, my five kids and I need to take any antibiotics for the throat infections. We never see any ENT surgeons in our whole lives, or need to be admitted to the hospitals or end up with the operations (tonsillectomy) for our sore throats either. I did not even check their throats because for me as long as they could drink water, their throats were either normal or did not have any significant abnormalities. I did not even check my own throat for a sore throat, because I firmly believed that it was not necessary.

It was also not a problem when I was working in one of the hospitals in Perak. Even if the patients had persistently high fevers with severe sore throats, we could just start the antibiotics. Rarely did we admit the patients with Acute Tonsillitis to the wards. Even though we had a resident ENT surgeon at that hospital, it was still difficult to refer a patient with a tonsillitis infection to him.

Usually, we would refer the patients if they have had more than six episodes of Acute Tonsillitis infections in a year. During these attacks, they would have had persistently high fever and difficulty in eating and drinking water. Even with these histories, we would still be given the appointments by the ENT Surgeon in 3 to 6 month's time. In addition, most of these patients did not end up with the operations (tonsillectomy).

Anyways, most of our patients at our clinics that complain of a sore throat would drink either warm or hot water. They would also take hot soups. They might feel much better after taking these hot water or soups because the heat would numb the nerves, but they would prolong the problems because the hot water or the hot soups would increase the throat inflammations.

Therefore, we have so many patients that came to our clinics complaining of sore throat that did not recover even after 3 or 4 weeks. Usually they have been to three or four different clinics and they were already given with two or three different antibiotics including the strong antibiotics for e.g. the Zithromax. By this time, they would usually request for a referral to the ENT Surgeon.

The problem is, whenever I checked these patients they would have normal temperatures and their throats were perfectly normal. These findings correspond to the recommendations given by the WHO where they recommend to not giving antibiotics to 90% of the patients with either the Acute Tonsillitis or Acute Pharyngitis.

Here is another problem. I find out early on when I just started opening my private clinics that it was easier to tell the patients that they had infected throat or tonsillitis and to give them the antibiotics than to say that their throats were normal and they just need to take simple medication with plenty of cold or iced water.

Some of the patients even claimed that they suffer from chronic tonsillitis infections for many years, and wanted me to check their throats. Even in these cases I found out that most of them did not have any enlarged tonsils or no tonsils at all. However, sometimes even these patients would end up with the surgeries (tonsillectomy) because they thought that their sore throat would not be resolved unless the doctors remove something from their throats.

Therefore, if you have a fever and a sore throat, together with other symptoms such as the coughs and stuffy nose, and the temperature is not persistently high for more than 3 or 4 days, the chances are, you are infected with the Common Cold or the Flu infections. In these cases, try to do the following advice:

1.   **Do not ask your doctor to check your throat.** It is the same with your kids. As long as you and your kids could drink water, don't ask your doctor to check your throat. I didn't check all my kid's throat either and they are very healthy now. The reason is that most patients that have their throats checked **would end up with the antibiotics.**

2.   **Don't take warm or hot water, or hot soups.** They would prolong the sore throat. Stop all of them and instead take cold water from the fridge, iced water, ice cubes or ice cream.

3.   **Don't take antibiotics.**

Drink Cold Water or Hot Water?

As I mentioned above, most Malaysians would take warm or hot water, together with the hot soups whenever they have a fever or a sore throat. Many other people also do the same, e.g. patients from the South East Asian countries, India, China and even from Russia (Yes, I have many patients from different nationalities at one of my clinics).

If you take warm or hot water, or hot soups, you will increase your body temperature and increase the throat inflammation. That is why in some patients do not recover even after 3 or 4 weeks of having the infection. The CDC, US in their 21 pages *'Flu homecare guidelines'*, are giving the the following recommendations: (https://www.cdc.gov/flu/pdf/freeresources/general/influenza_flu_hom ecare_guide.pdf)

1.   *Have **Cooler** or **pitcher with ice and drinks** in the room* (Page 8).

2.   Use a squeeze bottle or a straw for people too weak to drink from a cup. Or ***offer ice chips or frozen ice pops to suck on*** (Page 12).

3.   Treating sore throat: Offer the person - ***Ice chips or frozen ice pops* to numb the throat** and get fluids into the body (Page 20).

It is different if you want to take a shower or a bath while having a fever. In this case, you need to take a slightly warm shower or a slightly warm bath to prevent the sudden drop of your body temperature.

CHAPTER 9

COVID-19 AND OTHER INFECTIOUS DISEASES

'The environment is changing and so are the viruses.'

                   -       *Steven Magee*

COVID-19

The year 2020 has been a really tough year for us all. The Covid-19 infection, which started in December 2019 in Wuhan, China has caused havoc to the world. The infection rate is still not coming down even though initially we thought that it would disappear by the summer of this year. As of 9 October 2020, there were 36.7 million cases that had been confirmed worldwide, with more than 1.07 million deaths.

Covid-19 is caused by the corona virus. It is one of the viruses that cause the common cold infections. We always thought that the viruses that cause the common cold infections were not dangerous.

However, the corona virus has been very successful in changing or in mutating itself to become one of the most dangerous viruses that can cause the pandemic infections and cause many deaths as the Influenza A virus does. Unlike the Influenza A virus, the Covid-19 is also dangerous in the hot weather, and even more dangerous in the cold winter.

Corona Virus

The Corona viruses are named for the crown-like spikes on their surfaces. They are a group of RNA viruses that cause diseases in mammals and birds. Human Corona viruses (HCoV) were first identified in the mid-1960s. In humans and birds, they cause **respiratory tract infections** that can range from mild to lethal.

The mild illnesses in humans include the common cold infections, while the more lethal varieties can cause the Acute Respiratory Syndromes such as the SARS, MERS, and Covid-19. At the moment there are no vaccines or effective antiviral drugs to prevent or treat human corona virus infections.

There are seven strains of the Human Corona Viruses that can infect people, 4 would cause the Common Colds and 3 would cause the Acute Respiratory Syndromes.

The 4 strains of the Human Corona viruses that cause the Common Colds are HCoV-229E, HCoV-NL63, HCoV-OC43 and HCoV-HKU1.

The other 3 strains of the Corona viruses that cause the **Acute Respiratory Syndromes** are:

1.	SARS-CoV: causes Severe Acute Respiratory Syndrome (**SARS**).
2.	MERS-CoV: causes Middle East Respiratory Syndrome (**MERS**).
3.	SARS-CoV-2: causes Corona Virus Disease 2019 (**Covid-19**).

**A.	<u>Common cold</u>**

In humans, the virulence (the severity or harmfulness of the virus infection) of the Corona virus infection vary significantly. The 4 strains of the common Human Corona Viruses HCoV-OC43, HCoV-HKU1, HCoV-229E, and HCoV-NL63 continually circulate in the human population and produce the generally mild symptoms of the common cold as mentioned in the previous chapter.

These Corona Viruses cause about 15% of the common cold infections. They have a seasonal incidence occurring in the winter months in the temperate and cold countries. Whereas it can occur anytime of the year in the tropical countries.

**B.	<u>Acute Respiratory Syndrome (ARS)</u>**

As mentioned above, there are 3 strains of the Human Corona Viruses that cause the Acute Respiratory Syndromes. So far they have caused 3 major outbreaks since 2002, as described in Table-14 below:

1	Virus	SARS-CoV	MERS-CoV	SARS-CoV-2
2	Disease	**SARS**	**MERS**	**Covid-19**
3	Outbreaks	2002-2004	2012, 2015, 2018	2019-2020 Pandemic
4	Date of first identified case	Nov 2002	June 2012	Dec 2019
5	Location of first identified case	Shunde, China	Jeddah, Saudi Arabia	Wuhan, China
6	Age average	44	56	56
7	Confirmed Cases	8,096	2,494	36.7 M (9/10/2020)
8	Deaths	774	858	1.07 M
9	Case Fatality Rate	9.2%	37%	2.91%

Table-14: Characteristics of Corona Viruses Strains MERS-CoV, SARS-CoV and SARS-CoV-2.

a.   Severe Acute Respiratory Syndrome (SARS)

In 2003, following the outbreak of Severe Acute Respiratory Syndrome (SARS) which had begun in 2002 in Shunde, China and spread elsewhere in the world, the World Health Organization (WHO) issued a statement that a novel Corona Virus identified as SARS Corona Virus (SARS-CoV) was the causative agent for SARS. More than 8,000 people were infected, with about 9.2% of the patients died.

b.   Middle East Respiratory Syndrome (MERS)

In September 2012, a new type of Corona Virus was identified, initially called Novel Corona Virus 2012, and now officially named as the Middle East Respiratory Syndrome Corona Virus (MERS-CoV). As of December 2019, 2,468 cases of MERS-CoV infection had been confirmed by laboratory tests, 851 of them died. This give the mortality rate of MERS-CoV at 34.5%.

The WHO found later on that the virus did not easily pass from person to person. It appears that the virus had trouble spreading from human to human, as most individuals who were infected did not transmit the virus.

c. <u>Corona Virus Disease 2019 (Covid-19)</u>

In December 2019, a pneumonia outbreak was reported in Wuhan, China, which was traced to a novel strain of Corona Virus. It was named as 'Severe Acute Respiratory Syndrome Corona Virus 2' or SARS-CoV-2 by the International Committee on Taxonomy of Viruses.

The Wuhan strain has been identified as a new strain of Beta Corona Virus with approximately 70% genetic similarity to the SARS-CoV, hence the name given as the SARS-CoV-2. The virus also has a 96% similarity to a bat Corona Virus, and that is why the virus is suspected to originate from bats as well.

For the first time ever, a Corona Virus has caused a pandemic infection that created worldwide panic and chaos which resulted in travel restrictions and nationwide lock-downs in many countries. It spreads through the salivary droplets released when an infected person sneezes or coughs.

As with any other viral infections, there is no cure for Covid-19. Antibiotics is of no use for a viral infection. The best way to slow down the disease is by:

1.   practising social distancing i.e. limiting close face-to-face contact with others.
2.   protecting yourself by washing hands with water and soaps and using the disinfectant.
3.   not touching your eyes, nose or mouth with unwashed hands.
4.   practicing good hygiene standard like covering your mouth and nose when coughing or sneezing
5.   avoiding close contact with any sick people.

Most of the infected people experience mild to moderate breathing issues. Serious illness might develop in people with underlying chronic medical problems such as having the cardiovascular problems, hypertension, diabetes, chronic lung diseases, cancer and other immuno-compromised diseases.

<u>Other Infectious Diseases in Malaysia:</u>

To complete this chapter, I will write about two other infectious diseases in Malaysia that can be misdiagnosed as the URTIs. These infectious diseases are the Dengue Fever and the Leptospirosis.

Infectious Diseases are disorders caused by organisms - such as the **bacteria, viruses, fungi or parasites**. Many organisms live in and on our bodies. They are normally harmless or even helpful, but under certain conditions, some of these organisms may cause certain diseases to us.

After searching the internet for quite some time, Table-15 below shows the number of deaths in Malaysia due to the URTIs, Dengue and Leptospirosis infections for the year 2008 to 2017.

SER	YEAR	NUMBER OF DEATHS / SERIOUS INJURIES						
		URTIs		Dengue	Lepto-spirosis	Road Traffic Accidents		Drowning
		Common Cold	Flu			Deaths	Serious Injuries	
1.	2008	0	?	112	46	6,527	8,866	Average 700-800 /year
2.	2009	0	78	88	62	6,745	8,349	
3.	2010	0	10	134	71	6,872	7,781	
4.	2011	0	?	36	53	6,877	6,328	
5.	2012	0	?	35	47	6,917	5,868	
6.	2013	0	?	92	71	6,915	4,597	
7.	2014	0	?	215	92	6,674	4,432	
8.	2015	0	?	336	78	6,706	4,120	
9.	2016	0	?	237	52	7,152	-	
10.	2017	0	1	177	-	6,740	-	

Table-15: Number of Deaths / Serious Injuries due to URTIs, Dengue fever, Leptospirosis, RTAs and Drowning in Malaysia.

Source:1.https://magazine.scientificmalaysian.com/issue-12-2016/dengue-vaccine-dilemma-route-prevention-yet/ - for dengue deaths 2008-2015.
2.https://umexpert.um.edu.my/public_view.php?type=publication&row=NTE yMDU%3D - for Leptospirosis deaths 2008-2012
3. Road Traffic Accident in Malaysia: Trends, Selected Underlying, Determinants and Status Intervention. International Journal of Engineering & Technology 7(4.34):112. December 2018
4. The Rakyat Post: H1N1 Is Still Prevalent In M'sia: What You Can Do To Prevent It FromSpreading.(https://www.therakyatpost.com/2019/12/30/h1n1-is-still-prevalent-in-msia-what-you-can-do-to-prevent-it-from-spreading/)

I also put the number of deaths due to the Road Traffic Accidents (RTAs) and Drowning, and the serious injuries due to the Road Traffic Accidents (RTAs). By doing this, I hope we could look at these three infectious diseases from different perspectives.

For the Common Colds, we know that every year millions of Malaysians are suffering from the infections, but we don't have the exact figure. In general, they rarely cause any deaths to the patients. For the Influenza or Flu Infections, even during the Pandemic Influenza A/H1N1 infection in 2009 only caused 78 deaths in 2009 and 10 deaths in 2010. There was one death due to the Influenza A/H1N1 on 13 April 2017 in Terengganu. Apart from that, there were *no record of deaths* due to the Influenza or Flu infections in Malaysia.

The number of deaths due to Influenza or Flu Infections was much less than deaths due to drowning for example, which even in 2009 was about 10 times more than the Pandemic Influenza A/H1N1/2009. The deaths due to Road Traffic Accidents (RTAs) in 2009 was about 86 times more than deaths due to the Flu infections, or 8,600% more. Apart from that, RTAs also cause serious injuries to another few thousand other victims.

In conclusion, the Common Cold and Flu infections rarely cause any deaths, except for the Flu during the pandemic infections in 2009. Unfortunately a large number of Malaysians are really scared about them and end up with the unnecessary blood tests and other investigations, with the antibiotics or anti-viral medicine, or both and sometimes with unnecessary hospital admissions.

At the same time we don't give a second thought about deaths or major injuries due to the Road Traffic Accidents or Drowning, which are much more than the deaths due to the URTIs.

A.   **Dengue Fever**

Dengue fever is an infectious disease caused by a virus called Dengue Virus (DENV). They are carried by female mosquitoes mainly of the species Aedes Aegypti. There are five different types of the dengue virus, called serotypes. They are referred to as DENV-1, DENV-2, DENV-3, DENV-4 and DENV-5.

This disease is used to be called a "break-bone fever" because it sometimes causes severe joint and muscle pain that feels like bones are breaking. People get the dengue virus from the bite of an infected Aedes mosquito. It is not contagious from person to person. Therefore, you cannot get the infection by touching, kissing or sharing utensils with the infected person.

In a mild Dengue Fever, the patient would have the following symptoms:

1. High grade fever (>38 °C).
2. Severe headaches.
3. Muscle, bone and joint pain.
4. Nausea.
5. Vomiting.
6. Rashes.
7. Loss of appetite,
8. Feeling tired or have no energy.

The fever would be persistently high even during daytime or after taking the paracetamol tablets. In most cases, there will be no coughing, stuffy nose or having sore throat.

In a severe form of a dengue fever, which is called a *Dengue Haemorrhagic Fever*, it can cause severe bleeding especially from the nose, gums and internal organs, a sudden drop in the blood pressure (shock) and death. Signs and symptoms of a Dengue Haemorrhagic Fever are as follow:

1. All of the above symptoms.
2. Persistent vomiting.
3. Bleeding from the gums or nose.
4. Blood in the urine, stools or vomit.
5. Bleeding under the skin (petechiae).
6. Difficulty in breathing.
7. Severe abdominal pain.
8. Fatigue.
9. Irritability or restlessness.

10.   Cold or clammy skin (shock).

11.   Sudden drop in blood pressure (shock) and death.

In Table-16 below, we can see that **the mortality (death) rate** for a dengue fever is very low. Every year only about 0.2% of the patients infected with dengue fevers would succumb to their infections. Since there were many more patients with Dengue fevers who recovered on their own and did not go to the clinics or hospitals, the mortality rate would be much lower than 0.2%.

Therefore, not every patient that is infected with the dengue fever should be admitted to the hospitals. In the government hospitals, they tend **not to admit** most of the patients with dengue fevers, unless they have very low platelets level or they have signs and symptoms of bleeding.

<u>PERCENTAGE OF DEATHS DUE TO URTIS, DENGUE AND LEPTOSPIROSIS</u>

YEAR	NUMBER OF CASES AND PERCENTAGE OF DEATHS											
	Common Cold			Flu			Dengue			Leptospirosis		
	Cases	Death	%	Cases	Death	%	Cases	Death	%	Cases	D	%
2008	M	0	0	?	?	?	49,335	112	0.22	1,400	47	3.4
2009	M	0	0	14,912	78	0.5	41,486	88	0.21	1,423	62	4.4
2010	M	0	0		10		46,171	134	0.29	1,961	65	3.3
2011	M	0	0	?	?	?	19,884	36	0.18	2,268	55	2.4
2012	M	0	0	?	?	?	21,900	35	0.15	3,365	48	1.4
2013	M	0	0	?	?	?	43,346	92	0.21	4.457	71	1.6
2014	M	0	0	?	?	?	108,698	215	0.20	7,806	92	1.2
2015	M	0	0	?	?	?	120,836	336	0.27	8,291	78	0.9
2016	M	0	0	?	?	?	100,028	237	0.23	5,284	52	1.0
2017	M	0	0	?	1	?	83,849	177	0.21	-	-	-

Table-16: Number of Cases and percentage of Deaths due to the URTIs, Dengue and Leptospirosis in Malaysia. M=Million

In normal people, the platelet level is between 150,000 to 450,000 platelets per microliter of blood (or 150 billion to 450 billion of platelet cells per litre of blood). Some government hospitals will admit a patient with a dengue fever to the ward if the platelets level decreases to below 60,000 per microliter of blood. Whereas other hospitals might admit the patients with even lower level of platelets, for example lower than 40,000 per microliter of blood.

They will keep the patients in the ward until the platelets level increased to more than 60,000 per microliter of blood or higher. They would discharge the patients at this platelets level or after all the bleeding have stopped.

Case No. 30
Mr H,
A Dengue Haemorrhagic Fever.

One of our patients, Mr H was a 35 years old man who complained of a high-grade fever for a few days. He also had severe headaches, body pain, joint pain, lethargy or feeling tired, feeling nauseous and loss of appetite.

However, what was alarming was that he had bleeding from the nose and the gums. One of our doctors immediately referred him to the nearest General Hospital for a possible Dengue Haemorrhagic Fever.

This General Hospital charged their patients differently from other government hospitals. Their charges were much higher than the normal government hospitals, but still much cheaper than the private hospitals. After a few days at the hospital the charges had already increased to a few thousands ringgit. Since he could not afford to pay for these charges, Mr H requested for an *At Own Risk (AOR)* discharge from the hospital.

He came back to our clinic when I was working there. I found out that his platelet level was about 40,000 per microliter of blood when he was discharged from the hospital. He was still having the bleeding from his nose and gums. He should have still been kept at the hospital with that low platelets level and the bleeding. However, since he could not afford the hospital bill, and he requested for an AOR discharge, the hospital just obliged.

Whereas at the private sectors, I had many dengue patients that had the platelet levels of more than 200,000 or even 300,000 per microliter of blood but were still admitted to the private hospitals because they could afford the hospital bills.

Here are the **mismatch of the Health Resource Allocations,** where the people that need the urgent medical treatment but do no get them because they could not afford the bills, but the one that do not need them get the best treatment available.

B.   <u>Leptospirosis</u>

Leptospirosis is *caused by a bacterium called Leptospira interrogans*. Many animals such as rats, mice, cows, pigs and dogs carry this bacterium. They carry the bacteria in their kidneys. These bacteria will end up in the soil and water through their urine. Therefore, Leptospirosis is spread in the pee of these infected animals.

You can be infected with the Leptospirosis from:

1.   Freshwater (such as from a waterfall, rapid, river, flooded area, pool, canal or lake) or soil containing infected pee gets into the mouth, eyes or a cut – usually during activities like outdoor swimming, fishing or even having a picnic near the above freshwater or soil.

2.   Touching an infected animal's blood or flesh– usually from working with animals or animal parts.

It is very rare to get a Leptospirosis infection from pets, other people or bites. The infected people may not have any symptoms, but they can become carriers. **In most cases**, Leptospirosis is unpleasant but not life threatening, like a case of the flu. It rarely lasts more than a week.

However, about 10% of the infected people could have a severe form of the Leptospirosis and require hospitalization. In Leptospirosis, a patient could have similar symptoms and signs as the Dengue Fever. These symptoms and signs include:

1.   High grade fever (>38 °C).

2.   Severe headaches.

3.   Feeling Cold / Shivering.

4.   Muscle, bone and joint pain.

5.   Nausea and Vomiting.

6.   Jaundice (yellow skin and eyes).

7.   Abdominal pain.

8.   Diarrhoea.

9.   Rashes.

However, in severe Leptospirosis, the infection can lead to a life-threatening multi-organ failure characterized by the acute liver failure, nephritis (kidney inflammation), pulmonary haemorrhage (bleeding from the lungs), meningitis (infection of the brain meninges), and cardiac arrhythmia. These multi-organ failures could eventually lead to death.

The mortality (death) rate for a Leptospirosis infection is also low, as can be seen in Table-15 above. The mortality rate for the Leptospirosis in Malaysia was between 0.9% to 4.4% for the years 2008 to 2016.

The actual rate should be much lower than these rates since most patients recovered on their own and did not go to the hospitals. Since the majority of patients with Leptospirosis infections have only mild symptoms, the government hospitals also tend not to admit these patients.

However, the mortality (death) rate for the Leptospirosis is higher than the Dengue fever. The mortality rate for the Dengue Fever was between 0.15% to 0.29% for 2008 – 2017. Whereas for the Leptospirosis the mortality rate was much higher, between 0.9% to 4.4% for 2008 – 2016.

It means that you are between 3 to 29 times more likely to die from the Leptospirosis infection than the Dengue fever if you are infected with either one of these infections.

One of the reasons for these higher mortality rate is the delay in diagnosing the problems and the delay in giving the antibiotics to the patients with Leptospirosis.

As you can see above, dengue fever is due to a viral infection whereas Leptospirosis is due to a bacterial infection. Since the Leptospirosis is less common than the dengue fever, doctors tend to treat the Leptospirosis as a viral infection without giving the antibiotics. When they realise that the infection could be due to the Leptospirosis, it could already be too late.

Therefore it is very important for you to inform the doctors if you developed **a high fever after visiting a waterfall, rapid, river, flooded area, pool, canal or lake, or your work involve in working with animals or animal parts.**

Discussions

The most common diagnosis for a patient that complains of a fever with or without other symptoms like headaches, coughs, sore throat, nasal congestion or bodyache is either the Common Cold, the Flu infection, the Dengue Fever or the Leptospirosis infection.

As you can see in Table-15 above, even the total number of deaths due to all of these four infectious diseases combined were very low. If you take the year 2016 for example, there were only 289 deaths out of millions of patients. This gave a very low mortality rate.

I know that I am talking about deaths as statistic here. It is not a nice way of doing it but we have to be frank and honest about it, so that we could see the bigger picture. Death is inevitable, especially at the hospitals and we really need to face this fact.

No hospitals in the world could reduce the number of deaths at their hospitals to zero. If you take the Flu infections for example, even in the US they have more than 22,000 people die every year (see Table-11) due to the infections, compared to 0 death in Malaysia.

If you compare this 289 of deaths to the number of deaths due to the Road Traffic Accidents in 2016, where there were 7,152 deaths due to RTAs against 289 deaths due to the Dengue, Leptospirosis, Common Cold and Flu Infections combined. It meant that in 2016 you were 24.7 times or more than 2,400% more likely to die from the Road Traffic Accidents than to the Dengue, Leptospirosis, Common Cold and Flu Infections combined.

All of these 289 deaths in 2016 were due to the Dengue fever and Leptospirosis. Whereas there were no deaths due to the Common Colds or Flu infections. There were also no complications from both of these Common Cold and Flu infections either, which meant that all the patients fully recovered from the infections without any complications *(except if they develop pneumonia due to the Flu infection, but unfortunately we don't have these data).*

Therefore, the government hospitals and most of the private clinics rarely do any blood tests on their patients for the Common Cold or the Influenza infections. For them **the chances of patients dying from both of them are almost zero**.

Even for a Dengue fever or Leptospirosis infection, they do not want to do the blood tests or to admit everybody to the wards either, because the hospitals would easily be full with these patients as what happened in 2009 with the Influenza A (H1N1) pandemic infection. In the beginning so many worried patients swamped the hospitals, which made the government hospitals to just stop seeing the patients with the H1N1 infections, unless their conditions were very bad.

However, the private hospitals have their own laboratories, which allow them to do many of these tests immediately. If they do the blood tests for the Influenza virus for their patients that come with fevers and the results are positive, in theory yes, they can lead to other potential serious complications like pneumonia. So they tend to admit these patients for the treatment and for monitoring in the wards.

Since the symptoms for the Dengue fever and Leptospirosis are different if compared to the Common Cold and Flu Infections where they would have a high grade fever and do not have other common symptoms like coughing, sore throat or nasal complaints, we could pick up these infections easily. Therefore, we could easily order for early blood tests for them.

However, the problems are that the normal dengue fever can progress into a more serious condition of a Dengue Haemorrhagic fever in a very short period of time. Patients that are prone to get Dengue Haemorrhagic fevers are:

1.   Patient with repeated infections.
2.   Infants and small children.
3.   Pregnant women.
4.   The elderly (Age > 65 years old).
5.   Patients with compromised immune systems.

Our aim is to admit these patients to the hospital as early as possible. However, money can be an issue, as you can see in Case No. 30 above. Even though he was diagnosed with a Dengue Haemorrhagic fever early and already admitted to the government hospital with a low platelets level and bleeding, but he was discharged from the hospital since he could not afford the hospital bill.

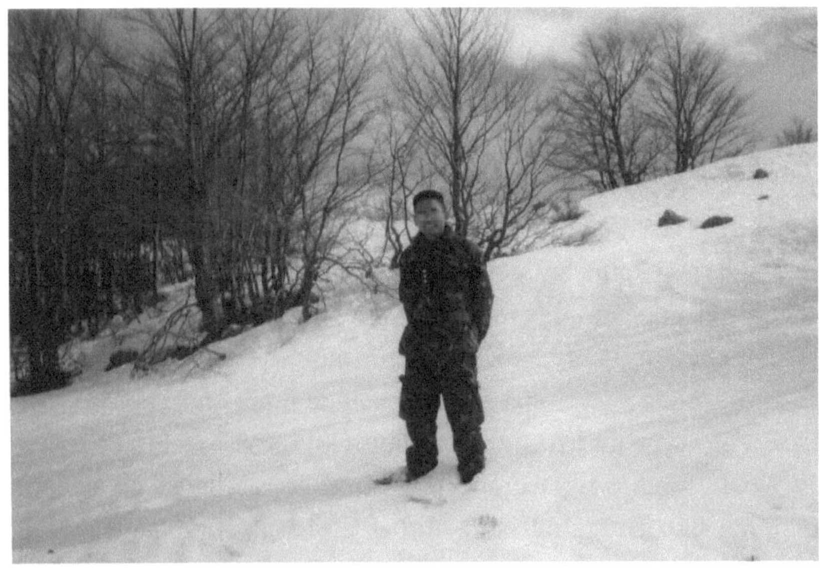

Picture-7: A Very Cold Winter in 1997, Bosnia-Herzegovina.

CHAPTER 10

TREATMENT FOR KIDS

'It is easier to build strong children than to repair broken men.'
-        *Frederick Douglass*

For most parents, their children are their life. They want the best of everything for their child. Money will not be an issue. These would include the medical treatment. If they think that their kids need that special treatment, then they want that special treatment to be given to their kids quickly. If these treatment require their kids to be admitted to the hospitals, they will make sure that their kids would be admitted to the hospitals as soon as possible.

This is the reason why it is very common to find a child that has been regularly admitted to the hospitals, especially to the private hospitals (since it is very difficult to get admitted to the government hospitals). Sometimes a 2 years old child would have been admitted to the hospitals more than 10 or 20 times, for various minor illnesses.

Some of them would end up with unnecessary procedures or even operations, whereas if the parents wait, some of these problems would heal by themselves. These would reduce the hospital admissions, procedures or operations, which in turn would reduce the chances of having complications from them.

These regular admissions to the hospitals for minor medical problems to me are wrong. Every time you kids are admitted to the hospitals, there will be more medication given to them. These medication are stronger too, including the intra-venous antibiotics, which go straight into their blood systems.

There would also be more tests and other procedures done to them. As in the Case No. 11 above, a girl with a simple Common Cold Infection ended up in the ICU. In the ICU there will be many strong medicine injected direct into your bodies. Your body would be connected to many different machines to act as artificial life support machines. Unfortunately she died in the ICU only a few days after being admitted to the hospital.

Apart from that, your kids will also be exposed to many different types of viruses and bacteria that are already present in the hospitals. Sometimes instead of being treated for the problems that they are being admitted for, they would need to be treated for the infections that they acquire at the hospitals.

These hospital acquired-infections would be stronger than the normal infections. Many patients have died from the infections that they get from the hospitals, for example the **Methicillin-Resistant Staphylococcus Aureus (MRSA)** bacteria, or other superbugs.

These bacteria became superbugs or became stronger bacteria because of the overuse of antibiotics. According to the Centres for Disease Control and Prevention (CDC), US, every year about 3 million people get sick from the superbugs, and about 35,000 die. *(Refer: https://www.nbcnews.com/health/health-news/dangerous-superbugs-kill-more-people-previously-thought-n1081086).*

Another wrong perception is that most parents think that their kids need antibiotics. They do not only believe that their kids need the antibiotics, but they need the strongest antibiotics available. This is again very wrong. In most cases, they do not need any antibiotics at all. That is why my kids were rarely given any antibiotics, sometimes not even once a year.

Those are the reasons why none of my 5 children has ever been admitted to any hospitals, privates or governments. None of them has been seen by any specialists either, except by the dermatologist for their acne problems. They also did not take any supplements or vitamins.

When they were young, we gave them one of the cheapest formula milk available in the market. The main reason for giving them the cheapest formula milk was that they could be found in any shops anywhere in Malaysia including in the small villages. Therefore, we did not have the trouble of running out of them.

(RPN: 50270)

LEMBAGA PEPERIKSAAN
KEMENTERIAN PENDIDIKAN MALAYSIA

(LP/KOM.6) Pin. 1/2013

SIJIL PELAJARAN MALAYSIA 2017

NAMA : ▮▮▮▮ BINTI ZUKI
NO. K/P : ▮▮▮▮
SEKOLAH : SMK TAMAN DESA

ANGKA GILIRAN : BGJ01A030
KOD DAFTAR : 8 JEN.DAHULU: 0

KOD	NAMA MATA PELAJARAN	GRED	
1103	BAHASA MELAYU	A	CEMERLANG TINGGI
1119	BAHASA INGGERIS	A+	CEMERLANG TERTINGGI
1223	PENDIDIKAN ISLAM	A+	CEMERLANG TERTINGGI
1249	SEJARAH	A+	CEMERLANG TERTINGGI
1449	MATHEMATICS	A+	CEMERLANG TERTINGGI
3472	ADDITIONAL MATHEMATICS	A+	CEMERLANG TERTINGGI
3756	PRINSIP PERAKAUNAN	A+	CEMERLANG TERTINGGI
4531	PHYSICS	A+	CEMERLANG TERTINGGI
4541	CHEMISTRY	A+	CEMERLANG TERTINGGI
4551	BIOLOGY	A	CEMERLANG TINGGI
2611	PENDIDIKAN SENI VISUAL	A+	CEMERLANG TERTINGGI

1119(GCE-O) - 1A
3756(LCCI) - 1
3756 PRINSIP PERAKAUNAN - A+ -LAYAK PENGECUALIAN ACCA-CAT-FA1
PERKARA ASAS FARDHU 'AIN - LULUS
LAYAK MENDAPAT SIJIL

PENGARAH PEPERIKSAAN

Picture-8: The SPM Result of My Vegetarian Daughter. She did not eat much when she was young and as a vegetarian now she even eats less than before. She was never seen by any paediatricians, or admitted to the hospitals, rarely given antibiotics and she did not take any vitamins or supplements.

The second reason was because we believed that there were not much difference between the cheap formula milk and expensive formula milk. As long as their stomachs were full, that was good enough. I knew a poor family who had never given any formula milk to their kids at all, but still all the kids managed to become doctors.

Yet all my kids were very healthy and very active at schools. They became prefects, English debaters, chess players, president of clubs or other council members, and they have started their own travelling trips. They also scored good results in their examinations.

My eldest child got 10 As (8A+s, 2As) in her SPM. She got a first class degree in Accounting and Finance from one of the universities in the UK. She has visited Mecca, Greece, Morocco, South Korea and about 15 other countries.

The third one got 11 As in her SPM (9A+s, 2As). Now she is doing a medical degree at the Newcastle University Medicine Malaysia (NUMED). The fourth also got straight As. He got 10 As in his SPM (4A+s,3As,3A-s) and the youngest child is still in the secondary school.

Another thing that I really noticed about my kids were that the one that got straight As in their SPMs did not like eating food. My third (girl) and fourth (boy) kids really hate eating especially when they were very young. I used to pay my fourth kid RM2 for every few bites of food that he ate.

It was not that I wanted him to eat. The problem was that I hate throwing away the food. Most of the time I would end up eating all those food. That was why I put on about 40kgs of weight after my marriage.

The third kid is much worse than the fourth one. Since both my wife and I were quite busy when we were young, she was taken care of by many different people including her grandmothers and a few different maids. I think she didn't like that and as a protest, she refused to eat. When she was a toddler, she was really thin and skinny you could easily mistook her for an African girl from a famine African country.

Even now at 20 years old she does not like eating. If she takes a late breakfast, she would skip her lunch, and dinner for her is always light. Recently she decided to become a vegetarian, which means that she even take less protein and fat than before.

Even with less eating, for a Malaysian she is taller than most girls. In fact, she is just slightly shorter than I am (and I am tall according to the Malaysian standards). She managed to get 11As in her SPM and is aiming to be a doctor one day.

A lot of parents are really worried that their kids are not eating well and not eating enough vegetables. Sometimes they requested their kids to be referred to the pediatricians for further check up because they are not eating well.

Some parents would even beat their kids for not eating food as they would have expected them to eat. Most kids are the same, they would only like to eat the food that they like to eat, nobody can force them to eat what they don't like to eat, but there are nothing wrong with them.

My advice to the parents, don't worry about your children who are not eating well. Just let them eat whatever they like, or don't force them to eat if they don't want to eat. You don't need to give them any vitamins or supplements either because in general whatever they eat already contain enough vitamins and supplements for their bodies. We only need a small amount of these vitamins and supplements.

In fact in Malaysia, most major diseases are due to over-eating, not under-eating. I know that we have many urban poor kids in the Klang Valley, in the East Coast of Peninsular Malaysia and in the East Malaysia.

They are the one that might need the vitamins and the supplements. Unfortunately they could not afford them, so these vitamins and supplements would end up to those who could afford but do not need them in the first place. If you want to do one thing for your kids, let them run around freely.

My second kid is a bit different. He was born with a few medical problems. He was born with an umbilical hernia, bronchial asthma, eczema and allergic reactions to certain food. He also had other simple problems, but more severe than the other kids.

If he had a diarrhoea, he could easily have 10 – 20 episodes of diarrhoea in a few hours. If he cried, he could easily cry for 2 hours non-stop. If he fell asleep after crying for 2 hours straight, and somehow we made some noises and woke him up, he could then continue crying for another one or two hours.

Our neighbours thought that we abused him because the amount of crying that he did. Even with these problems, he was never admitted to any hospitals and was never referred to any specialists either. The amount of medicine given to him were much less than the medicine given to any normal kids in Malaysia.

However, he missed many of his school days, as we believed that resting at home was part of the treatment, especially for his asthma. Even with these problems, he still managed to get As in English, Maths and Science for his SPM. Now he is in his final year at one of the university in England.

A.   <u>Umbilical Hernia</u>

For his umbilical hernia, the biggest size that it could get was about 3cm x 2cm in diameter, especially when he was crying. However, in babies with that size of hernia it seemed that it was really big and looked very scary.

Umbilical hernias appear as a bulge or swelling in the belly button area. We don't really know what the cause is. Most umbilical hernias don't need any treatment. Usually, the problem heals on its own by the time your child is 4 or 5 years old

So we waited, and true enough his umbilical hernia healed by itself before he even turned to one year old. Since the bulging could look very scary, some parents opted for an early operation. I had a baby patient at my clinic who went for an operation for his umbilical hernia, if I remember correctly at 8 days old.

When I saw him one day for other complaints, he was a few months old. I noticed that he had a big scar near his umbilicus. With that big scar, I think it could interfere with the normal growth of his abdomen. That is the reason why in some cases it is better to wait first rather than to go for invasive procedures straight away.

Another example involved my nephew who used to have many warts, hundreds of them all over his body. Since there were too many of them, the parents just left them alone. Fortunately, all the warts disappeared by the time he was in his late teens. There are no scars at all.

At my clinic, I had one girl who was about 5 years old. She had 4 warts over her back and arms. Her father brought her to the dermatologist, who used a laser to remove them. According to the father, it was very painful during the procedure that the girl cried and the doctor had to stop the treatment. The dermatologist managed to remove one of the warts, but left a big scar on the skin.

B.   <u>Allergic Reaction to Food and Eczema</u>

For his allergic reaction to certain food, we never did any blood tests to confirm that he had an allergic reaction or checked what type of food that he was allergic to. The main reason was that it was difficult to have a positive result that would help in finding the causative agents.

The second reason was that the results would not be 100% accurate, as you can see to what had happened in Case No. 1 above. We might end up with avoiding food that he was not allergic to, but kept giving him with the food that he was allergic to. Even if we found the food that cause the allergic reaction, the management would still be the same. Why would we want to do something that would not affect the way we treat the patient.

Many patients went for the blood tests to look for the things that they were allergic to. It sounds logical that if we find something that we are allergic to, then we can treat that allergic reaction or we could avoid those allergic agents.

The problem is the treatment for an allergic reaction is not that straightforward. There is no medicine that can cure the allergic reaction, except to treat the symptoms whenever you suffer from that allergic reaction.

It is the same in the US. They could not cure any patients who suffer from allergic reactions either. The problem is, in the US, in certain cases, some people would die from taking certain types of peanuts.

What they do is they would check and confirm that these people could develop severe allergic reactions to the peanuts. They would then be required to wear a bracelet, so that in the case of an emergency, the medical personnel would know that the problem is a severe allergic reaction, which can lead to an *anaphylactic* shock. The medical personnel could then immediately give the appropriate treatment.

Somehow, we were lucky. We found out by chance that he was allergic to egg yolk, or any food that contained egg yolk. If he accidentally ate these foods, his eczema would flare up and at the same time they could also trigger his asthmatic attack. Therefore, the first thing that we did was to avoid any food that contain egg yolk.

For his eczema, we applied plenty of moisturisers such as the baby oil or Vaseline. We only applied the steroid creams mixed with antibiotics whenever the attack was severe.

Too much steroid creams would cause the skin to become thin and dry, which in turn would make the eczema worse. Luckily, his allergic reaction to egg yolk and eczema were resolved when he was about 5 or 6 years old. Now we were left with his Bronchial Asthma.

C.   **Bronchial Asthma**

He had severe asthmatic attacks since he was about 6 months old and they almost disappeared when he was about 14 years old. The triggering factors for him was cold weather (for e.g. air-cond, raining for a few days or holidays in the Cameron Highlands or Genting Highlands), physical activities, food allergies and viral infections.

Since we knew that most of the infections were due to viruses, we rarely gave him antibiotics. Therefore, we were able to reduce the number of medicine that we needed to give to him.

For his asthmatic attacks we would give him 2 different inhalers such as the **V*entolin Evohaler*** and **S*eretide Accuhaler***. We would also give him another oral anti-asthmatic medicine (bronchodilators- medicine that cause widening of the bronchus, for e.g. Syrup Ventolin) and Syrup Prednisolone (steroid- strong anti-inflammatory medicine) at as low a dose as possible.

The treatment for the Bronchial Asthma is different now. We don't use the Short Acting β-agonist (SABA) inhaler such as the ***ventolin evohaler*** as much as before. The recommendation now is to use the combination of a Long Acting β-agonist (LABA) and Inhaled Corticosteroid (ICS) such as the **Symbicort Turbohaler**.

If the attack was due to a viral infection, then we need to add another 3 medicine, the paracetamol syrup for the fever, the cough syrup for the cough and the anti-histamines for the nose congestion. But to give 7 different medicine to a small kid was very difficult.

Therefore, to solve the problems we would reduce the number of times that we give the cough syrup and the anti-histamine to him.

By giving all of the above medicine, we managed to reduce the number of nebulisers given to him.

The reason for us not to give him the nebuliser was that we did not want to bring him out to the clinic every time we wanted to give the nebuliser. For sick kids to go out of the house was not that pleasant at all. Moreover, to go to the clinics or hospitals sometimes would be very stressful to the kids, which could make the attack worse or more severe.

D.　　Treatment for Kids

My other four kids were very easy to take care. They were born healthy without any medical problems. Since they did not have any asthmatic problems, they were never given any nebuliser treatment. Whenever they had acute URTIs, we only needed to give them the paracetamol syrup for the fever, and asked them to drink plenty of cold water and that was it. Sometimes we would also give the cough syrup, the anti-histamines for the flu and the anti-vomiting medicine, but since they did not like their tastes, they would refuse the medicine anyway.

While having the infections, usually they would refuse to eat any food. Once they have recovered from their infections, they would eat much more food than they would have normally eaten.

That is why I always advise the parents not to worry about their child not eating well, especially when they are sick. They won't have any appetite for the food, and sometimes eating would cause them to vomit, which would further aggravate their dehydration.

We rarely gave them other medicine for other simple complaints like diarrhoea, phlegm, poor appetite or stomach pain. My second child tend to have more severe form of other illnesses as well. For example, one day he had episodes of diarrhoea for more than 20 times in about 2 hours, and then slowly decreased in frequency.

Since he looked okay and was still active physically, I just gave him plenty of plain water. I used to have many parents requested their kids to be admitted to the hospitals because they had 4 or 5 episodes of diarrhoea in one day.

I also had many parents that came to my clinic requesting for nebulisers for their kids for having phlegm or coughing. Nebuliser is for an asthmatic patient, not for phlegm or coughing. There is no way that you can prove that your kids are having phlegm. For us phlegm is never a problem, so we never diagnose our kids as having phlegm problems, so we never give them any medicine for the phlegm.

Sometimes the parents requested their babies to have suction of their lungs done to remove the phlegm. I know that some doctors would agree to do that, but most of the time it's their teenager's clinic staff that would do that procedure.

For me suction should only be done at the hospitals, for example just after the delivery if necessary. Other than that, they rarely need the suction unless they are admitted to the hospitals with severe lung infections. That is why none of my kids has ever had suction done in their whole life.

E.   <u>**Common Cold with a sore throat- don't ask your doctor to check your kid's throat.**</u>

As in adult patients, most parents would ask their doctors to check their kids' throat, even though they did not complain of any sore throat. As I mentioned before, even with a sore throat you don't need to have your kid's throat examined. As long as he or she can drink water, it means the infection is not severe.

Just ask them to drink plenty of cold water, iced water or to take ice cream. If the sore throat is severe, give them paracetamol syrup as well. Even with a severe throat infection, only a small percentage of the kids require antibiotics, **most of the time your kids do not need any antibiotics at all.**

It is not easy to look into the kid's throats. Sometimes the doctors could not even see clearly because the kids would not be cooperating with the examinations. As I explained before, it would be easier for the doctors to just say that their throats are infected and to give them antibiotics rather than to say that the throats are perfectly normal and they do not need the antibiotics. This is even more common in adult patients, because most adult patients thought that since they had a severe sore throat, there must be something wrong with their throats.

Actually, **in most of the mild or moderate cases**, the doctors do not even need to examine your kids to diagnose the problems. If they have fevers with flu and coughs, the most common problems that they have are the simple Common Cold infections.

They just need to take simple medication like a paracetamol syrup for the fever, an anti-histamine for the flu and a cough syrup for the cough as I mentioned above. It does not matter whether the kids have a sore throat or not, **the aim is not to simply give the antibiotics**.

That is why I don't remember looking at my kids' throats when they were small. I did not even take their temperatures **unless the fever was very high**. Once they had the above problems, we would immediately gave them the paracetamol syrup and asked them to take plenty of cold water to bring down their temperatures and to reduce the throat inflammation.

When they were babies, we would regularly do a tepid sponging with wet cloth. Most of the time we did not even give the anti-histamines or cough syrups because most kids did not like taking these medicine, unlike taking the paracetamol syrup, which tasted nicer.

Yes, most of the time I treated my 5 kids who complained of fevers, coughs and flu with the paracetamol syrup and giving them plenty of cold water to drink. They worked most of the time if not all, as none of them had ever been admitted to the hospitals or needed to be referred to any specialists.

These treatment even worked for my fourth kid, whom would have had a very high temperature of 40-41°C whenever he had a fever. If I were not a doctor, I am sure that he would have ended up in the hospitals or in the ICUs, with the many complications that could arise from the treatment there.

Specialist Treatment and Hospital Admission for Kids

Some parents are proud that their kids are always treated at the famous private hospitals, always given the most expensive antibiotics or they have their own pediatricians. I beg to differ. I am proud that all my kids were never admitted to any hospitals, rarely take antibiotics and they were never seen by any pediatric specialists either, for the reasons that I mentioned above.

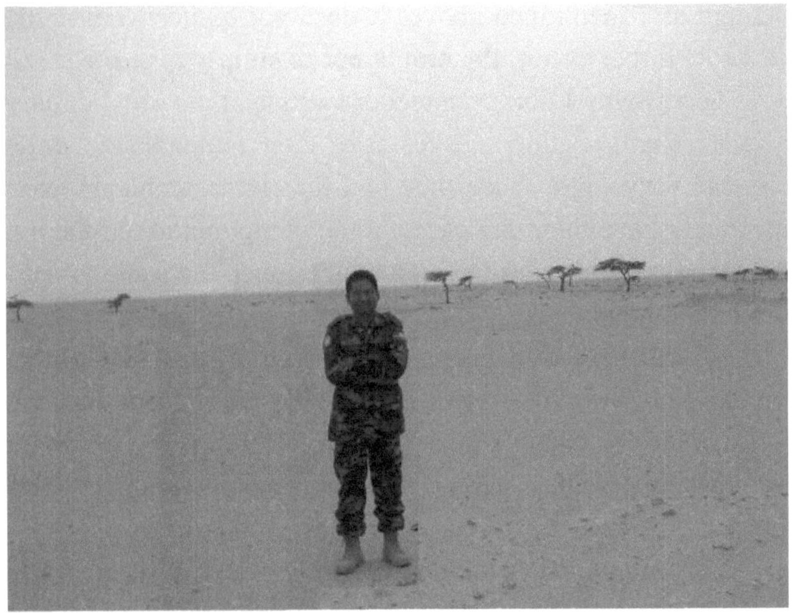

Picture-9: An Empty Sahara Desert.

CHAPTER 11

GOVERNMENT HOSPITALS VS PRIVATE HOSPITALS

'When I told the doctor about my loss of memory, he made me pay in advance'.

-Anonymous

The way the patients are treated at the government hospitals is very different from the way the patients are treated at the private hospitals. Both have their own advantages and disadvantages.

These differences in the managements have evolved on their own for many years, to become as what they are today. If we knew how both of these systems work, then we could use both of them at the same time to get the most benefit out of both systems.

Waiting Time

One of the differences is the waiting time between the patient registration and the treatment given. At the private hospitals the registration is very quick and straight forward, and you will be directed either to be seen by their medical officers at the out-patient clinics or emergency department, or straight to the specific specialists at the specialist's clinics.

If you are required to be admitted to the ward for further investigations or treatment, then you will be admitted straight to the ward, either through the out-patient clinics, the emergency department, or through the specialist's clinics.

At the government hospital it is a bit complicated. If you have a non-emergency medical problem for example, you need to go to their out-patient clinics at the 'Klinik Kesihatan' or District Health Clinic first. It is up to the doctor at the District Health Clinic either to treat you at the District Health Clinic, or to refer you to the specialist's clinics or to the hospital for the admissions.

Most of the government hospitals are very busy. They also have limited amount of resources. By asking the non-emergency patients to go to the District Health Clinics, the government hospitals can then focus their treatments for the emergency cases and for the chronic and more difficult to treat cases such as the patients with heart diseases, cancer, diabetes with complications, uncontrolled hypertension and many more.

Whereas the private hospitals are business entities. Their aim is to get as many patients as possible so that they can generate as much income as possible, like any other businesses.

Getting a Specialist Treatment

Because of this red tape, sometimes it takes a few months or even a few year for a patient that request or require a specialist's treatment at the government hospitals to be referred to the specialist doctors. Whereas at the private hospitals you can see the specialist doctor even on the same day.

At the private hospitals, everything is fast. Sometimes they can do all the investigations, procedures and even treatment on the same day. Whereas at the government hospitals, usually they take much longer time to do all these investigations, procedures or for the treatment.

Therefore it is not a surprise to see many people with the medical cards (usually provided by their employers) choose to go to the private hospitals instead of the government hospitals.

If we compare the speed of the treatment given by the government hospitals and the private hospitals above, we can say that the private hospitals are much better than the government hospitals. But for many of the medical problems that we suffer from, giving less treatment and letting our body to heal naturally give the same results, if not better.

     <u>MALAYSIAN PRIVATE HOSPITALS</u>

As I mentioned earlier, Malaysia has one of the best health care services in the world. There were almost 1 million medical tourists that visited Malaysia in 2016, more than 1 million in 2017 and the figure was expected to rise again in 2018. On average, the number of medical tourists have increased by 100% in the last five years. These patients were coming from Indonesia, India, Singapore, Japan, Australia, Europe, the US and the Middle East.

The fact that our medical tourism is expanding at a very fast rate every year for the past few years is a testimony that our private hospitals are being recognised as being excellent centres for the medical treatment.

The International Living publication also said that the health care available in Malaysia is not only much cheaper or at a more affordable price, but also sometimes even better than what are on offer in developed countries. These foreign patients generated a revenue of RM1.0 billion in 2016 and RM1.3 billion in 2017 on hospital charges alone to Malaysia.

Malaysia gains much more from the incidental spending outside of hospital fees, with patients and their families spending an estimated RM5.0 billion in expenditure on other things such as the transportation, hotel, food and shopping.

Even the UK does not have as many and as advanced private hospitals as Malaysia does. Small private hospitals in the UK would charge very expensive fees compared to the Malaysian Private Hospitals.

Most of the patients in the UK could not afford these expensive private hospital charges. Their other alternative is to go to the government hospitals i.e. the NHS even though they have private medical insurances and the queues are long.

Malaysia can also be proud of hosting some of the best-trained doctors in Asia if not in the world. The majority of them have undergone training in the United Kingdom, Republic of Ireland, Australia, New Zealand, Canada or the US. The English-speaking doctors have also minimized the language barriers between the patients, thus providing a significantly less stressful situation for the patients.

Another thing that I am personally proud of is that our private hospitals have become so efficient that they put other businesses to shame. At the private hospitals there is little to no waiting time when you arrive at the hospital. It is as simple as registering at the hospital of your choice and then waiting for that particular specialist to see you.

Even in the UK, it takes from a few days to a few weeks just to get an appointment to see their General Practitioners (GPs). In addition, it would be up to their GPs whether the patients should be referred to the specialists or not, even though they have a private insurance card. These GPs need to follow strict guidelines and procedures before they could refer their patients to the specialists. Then it will take months before their specialists will see these patients.

My Own Experiences at a Private Hospital Specialist's Clinic

To see a specialist doctor or a consultant at a government hospital is very difficult. Many people need to wait between 3 - 6 months, sometimes even longer just to be seen at a government's specialist clinic. Even at this clinic, you either need to see their Medical Officers or their Registrars first. These doctors would then discuss your problems with either their young specialists or if you are lucky with the consultants in that department.

After complaining of worsening eye problems for a few months, I asked my father to come down to Kuala Lumpur to see a private ophthalmologist at one of the private hospitals in the Klang Valley. He had been complaining of the pain and discomfort in both eyes in bright sunlight for a few years, but they were getting worse for the past several months. The problems were so intense that he needed to sleep in the afternoon so that his eyes were not exposed to the sunlight.

He was about 82 years old at that time, but for someone that had been very active physically throughout his life, he hated having to sleep during daytime. He was still driving his car and these eye problems also limited his driving activities. He arrived at my house late in the evening. The next day I brought him to the private hospital just near my house without an appointment.

The way our private hospitals work is that, you can just walk in to see any specialist during the working hours every day without any appointments. There will always be one or two specialists from that department that are available to see you. For the next appointments, you need to follow that doctor's schedule, unless you decide to change the specialists.

If you are using an insurance panel or a Third Party Medical Card (usually provided by your company), then you need to get a referral letter first from your general practitioner first. The reason they do this is to make sure that the reason for you to be referred to the specialist is genuine.

But in Malaysia in general most patients and doctors do not follow this rule. Most patients believe that it is their rights to get a referral letter immediately from their general practitioners even though they do not have any significant complaints, and most general practitioners do not want to argue for something that nobody would want to listen.

After waiting for about 20 to 30 minutes, my father was seen by a lady ophthalmologist. After introducing myself as a doctor (which means that she can explain everything straight to the point) and telling her about my father's problem, she did a few examinations on my father.

Once she finished with the examinations, she explained that what my father had was a permanent damage to some parts of the retina, either due to old age, smoking or other causes. There was no treatment for this problem and my father just need to adjust his lifestyle to his eye problems. That was it. In less than 1 hour I got the information that I needed to know about my father's problems.

Yes, I just needed that 1 or 2 minutes of explanation. It only cost me RM60.00 for the consultation. However, my father was still not satisfied. He asked another brother of mine to bring him to another ophthalmologist at another private hospital. Unfortunately, the finding was the same.

It also happened to my mother. One day she complained of passing out copious fresh blood in the urine for a few days. Since she did not have any pain during that time, we call the complaint as a *painless haematuria.* Painless haematuria is a major symptom especially in the elderly, and the first thing that we need to rule out is a bladder cancer. She was about 70 years old of age at that time. I immediately asked her to come down to Kuala Lumpur for either an urgent ultrasound scan or an appointment with a urology specialist.

When she arrived in Kuala Lumpur, I already arranged for her to have an ultrasound scan done at one of the diagnostic centres. An appointment with a urologist was arranged by my wife at her medical school. Since the diagnostic centre was a bit busy, we spent about 4 hours waiting before the ultra-sound scan to be done and the report to be completed.

As the ultra-sound finding was normal, we needed to cancel the urology appointment because a government urologist will usually refuse to see a patient that have a normal ultrasound of the bladder and kidneys. Since it was her first ultrasound scan in her life (at the age of 70 years old), I also arranged for her to have a complete ultra-sound scan of her abdomen and pelvis. Apart from the bladder and kidneys, the scan also checked my mother's liver, gall bladder, spleen, uterus, ovaries and for any abnormal mass in the abdomen. The total cost was RM240.00.

Now I do not have to worry about my mother having possible problems with her abdominal organs for the next 3 to 4 years. I treated her with drinking plenty of plain water and her problem resolved after a few weeks.

I also brought my brother's mother-in-law, Mrs C to go for the ultrasound scan together with my mother, since she was already in Kuala Lumpur at that time. She was about 67 years old and also never had any ultra-sound done in her whole life, I thought it was a good idea just to do an ultrasound scan for her abdomen.

Mrs C had many medical problems, including Hypertension, Diabetes Mellitus, Hypercholesterolaemia, Gout, Skin Problems and Back pain. She was managed at one of the district hospitals in Terengganu. She was taking 8 to 10 different tablets for her problems. For her back pain, it was treated as a simple musculo-skeletal pain with pain-killers, even though she was an elderly person, with diabetes and hypertension.

When the ultra-sound result came out, she was found to have a big kidney stone in her right kidney. The stone was at the opening of her ureter, which was starting to block the ureter and causing the right kidney to swell. Immediately I wrote a referral letter to the doctor in-charge of her other medical problems at that district hospital that she normally goes for her monthly check-up.

Since she was already in the system, the doctor at that district hospital immediately referred her to the Surgical Department, Kuala Terengganu General Hospital. About 3 months later, she already had a procedure done to remove the stone. This accidental finding should have cured her back problems. That was also her first time having an ultrasound scan done in her whole life.

Problems with Malaysian Private Hospitals, Private Clinics and Private Patients

As I mentioned earlier, not many people are aware that simple hospital procedures, operations or even a simple health screening can be very dangerous. Medication that we use at the hospitals are mostly drugs or chemicals, which have their own side effects. Apart from that, some of the medical procedures and operations done at the hospitals could have their own complications. Even a simple health screening has its own problems as I mentioned in Chapter 1 above.

A simple mammogram test could **over-diagnose** between **120-140 normal women** for every **10,000 women** that go for the tests in the UK, which could lead to the unnecessary treatment. Even my wife, who is a doctor, has never done any mammogram test in her whole life. She proudly told me that she would never do the mammogram tests, unless she has enough symptoms and signs that justify her to have a mammogram test. Why? Because she knew what exactly was going to happen. She would be **more likely to be over-diagnosed** than **to get the benefits from the test**.

In a study done in the US and published in the British Medical Journal (BMJ) in 2016 as I mentioned in Chapter 1 above, estimated that the number of deaths in the US in 2013 due to **iatrogenic complications** were about 251,000 deaths, or at 9.67% of the total death. This is a very high number of deaths that we should not take lightly.

In general, I am very happy with the services that are given by the private hospitals. However, two major factors totally change the whole scenario. These two factors are so significant that they change the whole concepts that are very good about these institutions.

It is like the presence of the winter season in the US and UK changes the whole characteristics of the Flu infection in these 2 countries if compared to Malaysia. The presence of the winter in the US and UK make them to have more than 22,000 deaths in the US and a few thousands deaths in the UK every year due to the Flu infection if compared to zero death in Malaysia.

These two factors are as follow:

1.   **<u>Business Entities.</u>**

    a.   Both the private hospitals (including the diagnostic centres) and private clinics are business entities. Even the government treats us like normal business companies. We are subjected to so many rules and regulations, and our income is taxed like any other business companies.

    b.   Once you are in the private sectors, there are many different government departments that you need to deal with. In general, all these rules, regulations and different departments that you need to deal with make your business more difficult and more expensive to run.

    c.   They also make our lives much more difficult. I knew that sometimes it takes a few years just for the government officer to approve one Operation Theatre (OT) at a private hospital or at a diagnostic centre. Some of the delays sometimes was due to a single word, for e.g. *bilik (room)* instead of *tempat (space)*. I really hope that the new government could change how the government servants perform their duties.

d.   Since we are doing business like everybody else, then our main goal is to get the most profit out of it. Nobody can blame us for this. If making profit is wrong than we should close all the banks, the big companies, the fast food restaurants etc. as well. Even with this aim in mind, I would say that **80% of the private clinics are struggling to survive**. As it happens, our former prime minister's premium bakery shops closed down their businesses without a single ringgit of profit after 13 years of doing business. (He not only did not get any profit, but lost most of his capital too).

e.   Therefore, with all due respect to all the specialists and doctors at the private hospitals and private clinics (to a lesser extent since they don't have expensive procedures or surgeries), their managements would be biased towards profit. There will be more of over-diagnoses and over-treatment in the private sectors if compared to the government hospitals. This is a sensitive issue and I think we should let the new government to handle it.

2.   Medical Cards / Private Insurance Companies- Private Patients Factors

a.   Many big businesses or companies cover the medical expenses of their employees. They cover either the full expenses or part of the expenses by giving their employees different medical cards, which have been agreed upon by these big businesses or companies.

b.   With these medical cards, their employees could go to the private hospitals, which they could have not afforded if they were to pay by themselves. Even though the cards are meant for them to go to the hospitals for genuine medical problems, sometimes they would try to use them even for minor medical problems or unnecessary medical procedures. They would feel that they were at a loss if they are not using the medical card's benefits given by their companies.

c.   Therefore, many employees would request or sometimes demand to be referred to the hospitals even for minor medical problems. Sometimes they do not even have any complaints at all but requested to be seen by certain specialists just in case that specialists could find something wrong with them.

d.   **To find something wrong in a normal person (i.e. doing a medical screening) is worse than to treat a patient with a known medical problem**. Now you have to do all the tests that are available on the market to rule out any possible diseases that a normal person could have.

e.   In fact, it would be more profitable for a private medical center to do a medical screening on a normal person than to treat a patient with a known disease. This is also a sensitive issue and I think it would be better for the new government to handle it.

f.   Private Insurance cards are also becoming more popular in Malaysia now. Some of the people who buy this insurance know the way to go around it. Once they are accepted by the Private Insurance Companies they would find ways to be admitted to the hospitals and go for many tests or procedures unnecessarily.

g.   All these unnecessary tests, procedures, or operations would increase the total expenditure costs to our health system, which in turn would increase the prices further in the future because these unnecessary demands keep expanding every year.

B.   <u>MALAYSIAN GOVERNMENT HOSPITALS</u>

To explain the way the government hospitals work is not that easy and straight forward. To make it simpler to understand, I would need to compare this system with how the other government departments work first. I will write about my own experiences in dealing with two of these establishments before I write about the way the patients are managed at the government hospitals.

a.   <u>**Applying a Business Loan at a GLC bank.**</u>

When I left the military service in 2009, I immediately opened three private clinics as the majority shareholder and bought another minority shares at another clinic, using a franchise system from one of the biggest primary care provider in Malaysia. I also opened a medical shop with another partner selling over the counter medicine, disposable medical items and medical equipment. **Yes, I had been dreaming of becoming a big businessman since I was a teenager.**

Since all these businesses were new, we collected a certain amount of money as our initial capital, hoping that the income produced from the daily earnings can cover the rest. However, in business I can confidently say here that nothing that you have ever imagined happened would happen. The profit that you have imagined could easily be made was the last thing that could have ever been materialised. So many other things could have gone wrong first, which would make your business to fail before you could ever see your first ringgit of profit.

The same thing happened to our previous prime minister's business, where after 13 years he had to close down his premium bakery business without even a RM1 of profit. It is not only that, most probably he would have lost all his capitals or investments that were invested into the business, which ran into many millions of ringgit. *(Ref:1.http://cppwealth.blogspot.com/2011/07/mahathir-yet-to-make-money-from-loaf.html.   2.https://www.nst.com.my/news/nation/2018/04/356887/dr-mahathirs-loaf-closes-down)*

At the same time, he would also have many other bank loans and company debts to pay. He said in one of his speeches that in business, if you thought that you need RM1 million for your business, then you need at least 3 times of that amount of money just to make the business survive. He said further, "I have put in more money in the company but I have got nothing".

The same thing happened to me, our initial capital only lasted for about three months. Then all the shareholders had to inject more money into the clinics and shop every 2 to 3 months. In addition, to make matter worse, I got very little money as a salary or sometimes none at all, as all the businesses were not doing well. I had to use most of my savings and my gratuity money that I got when I left the military.

I also had to sell four of our houses (3 of my houses and 1 of my wife's house) either to cut down our expenditures, which meant that we sold the houses at a loss, or to get some money so that I could inject them into the businesses.

Anyways, since I have exhausted all of my money, my savings, and sold all the houses that can be sold (I have another house that I bought in a northern state that is now worth less than 5% of the original value, and I am still paying about RM1,400.00 every month for the bank loan for the next 20 years), the next step was to apply for the business loans or personal loans from the GLC companies that were given hundreds of millions of ringgit or even billions of ringgit by the government to help people like me, an SME businessman.

To cut it short, I wished I could have just gone to one of these banks or companies and be treated the way a lot of patients are treated at the private clinics or hospitals. I wish I could just see their officers, give my IC and my business registration certificate and ask them to refer me to their consultants or directors that can immediately approve the loan.

I would then immediately get the money to be injected into the businesses. This is not their money anyway, this is the money that is given by the government to be given as loans to business people like me. Once the loan is approved, the money will become my money, and I have to pay for every cent of it, plus interests. I do not use somebody else money.

But that was never happened. What happened was that I could not even pass the first officer. They wanted me to prove that I had a lot of money at the time when I was applying for the loan, and for at least

6 months to one year before that. I needed to prove to them that my cash flow was very good for at least the past 6 months to one year, and my businesses' cash flow were also very good for the last 6 months to one year.

They wanted proof as well in the form of so many documents that I needed to submit to them. Why did they want me to prove that I have a lot of money for them to give me their loans? The reason I applied for the loans was that I did not have enough money.

This is not fair. If a businessman talks about his or her business cash flow, it's the same like a patient talking about a life-threatening medical problem. This is not about a simple headache, or a neck pain, or a fainting attack. But somehow they don't want to listen to us but expect us to listen to them when they come to us with a simple headache and expect us to treat them like they have a life-threatening medical problem.

However, this difficulty of getting a loan is not a problem to me. For me it is a blessing in disguise, because in business, many people would have gone bankrupt by having too many loans to repay. The aim is to have as little loans as possible. But the problems in the medical world, most patients do not know that they are paying a lot of money for unnecessary medical procedures, treatment or operations.

Tan Sri A as in the Chapter 1 above would have paid millions of ringgit for his treatment and operations and wasting more than 15 years of his life before he realised that what he was doing was 100% unnecessary. I would easily say that about 60-90% of the patients that I referred to the private specialists or private hospitals in Malaysia were unnecessary. If I were to refer these cases to the hospitals in the UKor the Republic of Ireland, they would have refused to accept these patients.

Anyway, the bank officers would use many checks and balances before they could approve the loans. They would also use many other reports such as the CTOS and CCRIS as well as the internal bank evaluation before they could approve them. By doing these they hope that they would give the loans to the right person for the right reason and that person has the highest chance of repaying the loan. Even with these check and balance systems, about 20,000 Malaysians are declared bankrupt every year due to the bank loans.

The government hospitals have similar systems like these GLC banks before they could admit or treat their patients. One of the main reason is because they have limited resources. They have these systems so that the hospital admissions are for the right patients, at the right time and for the right reasons. The private hospitals could not apply these same systems, otherwise they would become bankrupt in no time at all.

b.   **<u>GST</u>**

All my clinics were not subjected to the GST as health services was one of the businesses that was exempted from this tax. However, not my shop, which was selling over the counter medicine, disposable medical items and medical equipment. This business was not making any profit, and we were really struggling with our negative cash flow. When the GST was introduced, everybody was afraid of being penalised with fines if we did not comply with this ruling, as we were reminded by this government department over and over again.

Our accountant advised us to register first with the custom department for the GST payment. However, our total income was never above the RM500,000 per year for us to be subjected to the GST payment. In addition, we never charged the 6% GST to our customers for a few reasons: we did not have any extra staff to do that, we did not know how to do it and we did not have time to do it.

Anyway, according to the custom officers, since we had registered our company with the GST system, we would still have to pay the 6% GST to the custom department regardless of the income that we got every year, even if it was less than RM500,000. We were paying this GST since the first day of the GST system being implemented. However, one day they came to our shop for a spot check and fined us another RM10,000 for a non-compliance to the GST.

Here was a company that had been struggling since the beginning, we did not get even a single cent out of this company. It is not only that, we also did not get a single cent from the capital that we injected and not a single cent for our salary. We had been paying the GST even though we were not supposed to as our income was always less than RM500,000 per year, and yet they still wanted to fine us for non-compliance to this GST.

No wonder; this was one of the reasons that brought the whole government down. The new Prime Minister, who was also affected by this ruling for his businesses, almost immediately canceled this GST system or brought it down to 0%, because it caused so many problems, difficulties, and hardships to the Small and Medium Enterprises (SMEs).

However, we had nobody to complain to at that time. The customs department did not want to listen to us, except that they kept threatening us with possible fines if we did not pay for the GST. Our government hospitals also practice the same system as the GST system. They are so many rules, regulations and red tapes that make getting treatment at the government hospitals so difficult.

Again how I wished that they could practice as what our private clinics and private hospitals practice. I can just drop at their offices, request to see their directors or bosses, and ask them for our shop to stop paying the GST, as our income did not meet their criteria for paying the GST, and everything would be settled immediately.

But nobody wanted to listen to us, like how the private doctors would listen to their patients. When patients requests for an MRI test for their back pain of 2 weeks, or to see an orthopaedic consultants for urgent appointments for their back pain, they would almost immediately get them.

At the private hospitals, all the doctors and the consultants there are always good listeners, and they will immediately have many tests done for whatever their patients have complained. Before you realise it you might have even ended with an operation or 2 to correct your backpain.

When I started my houseman training about 25 years ago, I chose the least busy hospital in Malaysia. As that hospital was in my home state, it made the choice even easier. I knew at that time that some hospitals in Kuala Lumpur, Selangor and Johor were really busy, where you didn't even have time to go to the toilets, especially during your 30 - 34 hours of on-call days.

Even today these hospitals are still very busy, and even the specialists go back late or stay at the hospitals when they are on-calls. They also have their own limited budget to be spent on patients for the whole year. Because of that, they really do not want to just simply admit any patients or perform any procedures unnecessarily. **And they are very good at this.**

That is why they don't just simply admit any patient especially the non-emergency cases. As most of the medical problems are non-emergencies, it seems that the government hospitals are treating most of their patients at the clinics or at the emergency departments, and let the patients go and rest at home.

The non-emergency problems include the common complaints such as the headaches, migraines, dizzy spells, fainting attacks, neck pain, back pain, stomach pain, heartburns, bodyache, tiredness and many more. They knew from their experiences, from the statistics and from the best practice guidelines that most of these patients did not require any hospital managements.

The best practice management for these patients are what we call the simple conservative treatment. These patients would be given simple medication like pain-killers or muscle relaxants, massage creams, medicated plasters, braces or nerve tablets for the back pain. pain-killers for the headaches and the paracetamol, cough syrup, anti-histamines and lozenges for the acute upper respiratory tract infections (URTIs) and so on.

They would then advise their patients to rest at home, so that their own bodies could heal themselves. The best place for the patients to rest and let their bodies heal themselves is at their home, not at the hospitals unless the patients are not stable.

Even if you give active and invasive treatment like epidural steroid injection or back operations for the back pain for example, or stronger medication including the intra-venous medicine for all these problems, the outcome could still be the same, but with more possible complications from these invasive treatment.

In the emergency cases, the treatment are different. The way the emergency cases are treated at the government hospitals are the same like how most of the patients are treated at the private hospitals. Say for example that you are diagnosed with an acute appendicitis, you would be immediately admitted to the surgical ward, have blood and urine tests done and would be booked for an urgent operation, the same way as you would be treated at the private hospitals.

In general, government hospitals tend to under-diagnose their patients' medical problems and under-treat their patients. Again, these are sensitive issues and we should let our new Health Minister and new government to do something about them.

CHAPTER 12

SIMPLE MEDICINE- 3 MINUTES MANAGEMENT
(SM- 3MM)

A Short History of Medicine

2000 BC: Here, eat this root.

1000 AD: That root is heathen. Here, say this prayer.

1860 AD: That prayer is superstition. Here, drink this portion.

1920 AD: That portion is snake oil. Here, take this pill.

2000 AD: That pill has many side effects. Here, take this root.

-   Anonymous

I am going to call the treatment that I am going to promote here in this book as a *'Simple Medicine-3 Minutes Management' (SM-3MM)* method. I will call it with another name once I can think of a better or a more elegant phrase. However, now I will just stick to the Simple Medicine- 3 Minutes Management, or SM-3MM in short.

This is a very crude method of predicting what treatment should you get for a particular medical problem. Even without this crude method, my experiences with the military hospitals, the government hospitals and the hospitals in the Republic of Ireland and the UK, they were much more stricter and much more conservative with the treatment that they were giving to their patients compared to my SM-3MM method.

Anyway, I am claiming here that it will only take about **3 minutes** to know how to manage some of your medical problems. I have explained in the previous chapters how a few common medical problems were treated in the military and at the government hospitals. In this SM-3MM method, you just need to answer a few questions that are relevant to your medical problems to know what are the best managements for them.

A.   <u>SM- 3MM METHOD: BACK PAIN / BACKACHE</u>

Say that you are working in your big office, which involves sitting for a long time and looking at the computer, or you are doing your normal activities such as walking, turning around or lifting objects from the floor. Suddenly you have a severe back pain, either in the neck area or lower down near the buttock. However, you can still continue with your work or your activities with no other complaints such as passing out blood in the urine etc.

If you want to know what type of treatment you should be getting for your back pain, you just need to ask yourself a few questions. No, you don't need to see a doctor to ask these questions, you can just ask these questions yourself. These questions are:

1.   Were you involved in a plane crash?

2.   Did you fall down from a 1,000 feet high building or an aircraft?

3.   Were you involved in an accident that made you bed-ridden for a few months?

4.   Does your back bone look curved or bent if seen from behind when you are bending over?

There you are, four simple questions that you should ask yourself for your back pain. All these four questions relate to the previous cases that I told in the earlier chapters. All of these four questions cover most of the possibilities that might have caused any damage to your backbones, muscles or nerves. I know that it is a very crude way of managing a medical problem. But if it works, than you could save a lot of money, time and the possibility of having complications from doing unnecessary tests, procedures or operations.

I am sure that you will only need to take 1 or 2 minutes to read the above questions and a couple of seconds to answer them. You don't even need the full 3 minutes to manage your back pain problem.

If your answers are NOES to all of the above questions, which usually are in most of the back pain cases that I see at my clinics, then the treatment for you is simple. Yes, I would say that in 98% to 100%

of cases you just need a simple treatment (I leave another 0-2% for possible rare cases, which are, very rare).

You just need a simple pain-killer for eg. the Non-Steroidal Anti-Inflammatory Drugs (NSAIDS), bed rest for a few days (not too long) until the pain gets much better or more bearable, and a few other things if you choose to use them, for examples the massage creams, medicated plasters and braces for your back.

The NSAIDS are also known as pain-killers or muscle relaxants. The problem is some patients would refuse the medicine if the doctors call them pain-killers. However, they would take the same medicine if we call them the anti-inflammatory drugs or muscle relaxants.

Then if you want to confirm about your back problems, you should go to your **regular** *Doctor or General Practitioner (GP)* and ask a direct question such as "will you (the doctor) go for further tests if you have the same back problem"? What you should not do is to google the internet about the back pain, and go to the doctor saying "I have a back pain and I think I need to do an MRI or I need to see an Orthopaedic Surgeon, can you refer me to the hospital?"

Even if all the answers are YESES, you still have a 95-100% chance of being treated with a simple treatment like Captain A, Commando A, Corporal A and Patient A in Chapter 6 were treated (again I leave another 0-5% for possible rare causes, which are again, very rare). However, if you have one YES answer or more, then you should go and see your GP for an examination. In fact, if you have any YESES answer to the above questions you have a 75% chance of already being admitted to the hospital.

No, you don't need to have any Neck x-rays or Back x-rays or Lumbar-Sacral x-rays, CT-scans or MRIs done for your backache. In most cases you also do not need other investigations such as the blood tests or urine tests either.

As with the back pain cases in the previous chapter, even **a fighter pilot, who was diagnosed with multiple levels of Slipped Discs, who used to be involved in vigorous and strenuous physical activities for many years, who flew fast jets with high-G force that**

act along their back bones, and then was involved in a plane crash still ended up with a simple treatment like I mentioned above.

Or like the Commando A, who had an almost free fall from a 1,000 feet high moving aircraft with multiple crack fractures of his back bones, was also given a simple treatment. I want to stress again, here we are talking about a fighter pilot and a commando, two of our most elite soldiers, who are very expensive people to train and take many years for them to become what they are, but still they got simple treatment for their backache. **The reason is that that is the best practice for managing the back problems.**

How about other diagnosis such as a cancer or other dangerous problems that might have caused the backache? Isn't it a good idea to have either a CT-Scan or an MRI done to rule out all these possibilities? The problem is, there is no magic in Medicine.

In most cases, you cannot just simply have rare diseases or rare cancer in your back bone, or in any other places for that matter. The probability or chances of anybody to have that possibility is very small, which make it necessary for you to have other specific signs and symptoms that suggest these problems first before we start doing the tests.

In theory yes, you can have these rare diseases, but the probability or the possibility of having that diseases are very, very small. Its like buying a lottery. Even though there is a chance that you would become very rich by buying a lottery, the truth is, this chance is very small, and most of the lottery buyers would lose their money instead of winning the money.

All doctors knew about this. If the chances are high, then most doctors will have MRIs done on themselves first, then on their wives, and then on their children, and then on their parents and so on and so forth. But the truth is, most doctors won't do that. That is what happened to Tan Sri A, who was thought to have a very rare cancer, but turned out to be normal. Unfortunately, he ended up with 3 unnecessary operations.

When you do any tests including the MRI, in most cases there will be some abnormalities found in your MRI reports (i.e. suspicious findings even though your body is normal). These abnormalities for the MRI of the back could be in the form of degenerative disc disease, old fractures or other suspicious findings. These findings are not Slipped Discs, but for most of these patients, they would still think that there is something wrong with their backbones. Somehow, their backache will not go away, but instead become more frequent because of these findings.

How about in patients with confirmed Slipped Discs in their MRIs in the private set up? For most of these people with confirmed Slipped Discs in their MRI tests, they would immediately think that there are having a dangerous disease in their backbones. Because of these thought, they would have more frequent back pain if compared to not knowing that there is something abnormal in their back. These type of people would easily end up with further treatment like the steroid injections or even operations.

CHOOSING WISELY RECOMMENDATIONS FOR BACK PAIN

1.   FOR DOCTORS
(Source: Go to "https://www.choosingwisely.org/. Click at 'Clinician Lists', then write 'back pain' in the keyword box and click 'Search'. You will get the advises as below.)

a.   *American Academy of Family Physicians*. Don't do imaging (i.e. X-rays, MRIs, CT-scans or other advanced imaging) for low back pain within the first 6 weeks, unless red flags are present.

b.   *American Academy of Physical Medicine and Rehabilitation*.

(1).   Don't order repeat epidural steroid injections without evaluating the individual's response to previous injections.

(2).   Don't order an EMG for low back pain unless there is leg pain or sciatica.

(3).   Don't order an imaging study (i.e. X-rays, MRI CT-scans or other advanced imaging) for back pain without performing a thorough physical examination.

c.   _American Academy of Neurological Surgeons and Congress of Neurological Surgeons._

(1).   Don't obtain imaging (i.e. X-rays, MRIs, CT-scans or other advanced imaging) of the spine in patient with non-specific acute low-back pain and without red flags.

(2).   Don't do an MRI scan of the spine or brain for patients with only peripheral neuropathy (without signs or symptoms suggesting a brain or spine disorder).

d.   _North American Spine Society._

(1).   Don't recommend bed rest for more than 48 hours when treating low back pain.

(2).   Don't use electromyography (EMG) and nerve conduction studies (NCS) to determine the cause of axial lumbar, thoracic or cervical spine pain.

(3).   Don't use Bone Morphogenetic Protein (BMP) for routine anterior cervical spine fusion surgery.

(4).   Don't recommend advanced imaging (e.g. MRI) of the spine within the first six weeks in patients with non-specific acute low back pain in the absence of red flags.

e.   _American Society of Anaesthesiologists- Pain Medicine._ Avoid imaging studies (MRI, CT-Scan or X-rays) for acute low back pain without specific indications.

2.   **<u>FOR PATIENTS</u>**

(Source: Go to "https://www.choosingwisely.org/. Click at 'For Patients', then write 'back pain' in the keyword box and click 'Search'. You will get the advises as below.)

a.   Back Pain is a common reason to see a doctor. There are many different tests and treatment for back pain. **_Some of them may not be right for you._** That's why it is important to talk to your doctor. Here are some things to consider before you have any tests or treatment.

(1). **Imaging Tests**. *You may not need them for back pain.* If you have back pain, your doctor may order an imaging test, such as an X-ray, a CT scan or an MRI. You might not need these tests, unless you have had back pain that doesn't get better after a month or two.

(2). **Some Imaging Tests Use Radiation**. X-rays and CT-scans expose you to radiation. The more scans you get the more radiation you get. This increases the risk of cancer.

b. **Steroid Injections**. Think twice before you receive additional steroid injections. People with back pain sometimes get a steroid shot in the spine. The shot can help reduce swelling and pain, especially if you have back pain from a pinched nerve. Your doctor may want to give you two steroid shots. But try to wait before getting a second shot. Wait to see if the first shot works. Then check in with your doctor. And consider other treatment as well. Multiple shots of steroids have risks such as:

(1). Raised blood pressure.
(2). Raised blood sugar levels.
(3). Prone for you to get sick.
(4). Weight Gain
(5). Lower Resistance to infection.

c. **Bed Rest for a Lower-Back Pain**. Think twice before getting more than two days of bed rest. There is no good evidence that long periods of bed rest help lower-back pain. In fact, studies show that patients actually feel better faster if they are active. Get an exam before getting more bed rest. Before you get more than two days of bed rest, your doctor should evaluate you. An exam is especially important if you have serious symptoms, such as:

(1). loss of bowel or bladder control.

(2).   fever.
(3).   numbness in your groin.
(4).   weakness, falling, or the inability to walk.
(5).   night-time pain.
(6).   new numbness, tingling, or sensory loss.
(7).   unusual weight loss.

B.   SM-3MM METHOD: HEADACHES, MIGRAINES, DIZZY SPELLS, VERTIGOS AND FAINTING ATTACKS.

Again, say that you suddenly have a severe headache, a migraine attack, a dizzy spell, a vertigo or a fainting attack, and you knew that you never had a high blood pressure, diabetes or other chronic diseases before, then you just need to ask 4 questions to yourself. It doesn't matter whether your headaches, migraines or your dizzy spells is only affecting the left side of your head, the right side, or any other sides. These 4 questions are as follow:

1.   Did you pass out for more than 8 hours with the headache, migraine attack, vertigo or dizzy spell?

2.   Do you feel the need to bang your head to the cement walls?

3.   Were you involved in a road traffic accident or other incidence that makes you have difficulties in talking, walking or seeing things?

4.   Do you have high temperatures with eyes discomfort or pain when looking at bright lights? (to rule out an infection in the brain).

If the answers are NOES to all of the above questions, which usually are in most of the cases that I see at my clinics, then the treatment for you is simple. You just need to take either 2 tablets of paracetamol 3 or 4 times a day, or simple pain-killers, and rest for 1 or 2 days if it is necessary. You don't have to go for a skull x-ray, or a CT-scan or an MRI of the brain. If there is one YES answer or more, you can still be treated with a simple treatment as mentioned above.

<u>**CHOOSING WISELY RECOMMENDATIONS FOR HEADACHES, MIGRAINES, DIZZY SPELLS, VERTIGOS OR FAINTING ATTACKS**</u>

1.   **<u>FOR DOCTORS</u>**

   a.   *<u>American College of Radiology</u>*. Don't do imaging (i.e. X-rays, MRIs or CT-scans) for uncomplicated headaches.

   b.   *<u>American College of Emergency Physicians</u>*. Avoid CT-scan of the head in asymptomatic adult patients in the emergency department with a syncope (fainting attack), insignificant trauma and a normal neurological evaluation.

   c.   *<u>American Academy of Neurology.</u>* Don't perform electroencephalography (EEG) for headaches.

   d.   *<u>American Association of Neurological Surgeons and Congress of Neurological Surgeons</u>*. Don't routinely obtain CT-scan of children with mild head injuries.

2.   **<u>FOR PATIENTS</u>**

   a.   **<u>Treating Migraine Headaches</u>**

   (1).   ***What drugs are good for migraines?*** If you have migraine attacks, try one of the drugs listed below. They all work best if you use them when the migraine is just beginning.

   (a).   Start with an Over The Counter (OTC) or non-prescription pain drug that combines aspirin, acetaminophen *(paracetamol)*, and caffeine (Excedrin Migraine, Excedrin Extra Strength, and generics). Or try *Non-Steroidal Anti-Inflammatory Drugs (NSAIDS)* such as ibuprofen or naproxen. *(NSAIDS medicine are commonly used in Malaysia for headaches i.e simple pain-killers).*

   (b).   If these drugs do not help, or your headaches are more severe, try one of the prescription migraine drugs called triptans, such as a sumatriptan (Imitrex and generic).

(2). ***Limit the use of all pain medicine.*** Do not use prescription pain medicine for headaches for more than nine days in a month. Do not use non-prescription pain medicine for more than 14 days in a month.

b. <u>**Imaging Tests for Headaches**</u>

(1). *When do you need a CT scan or an MRI- and when do you not?* CT scans and MRIs are called imaging tests because they take pictures, or images, of the inside of the body. Many people who have very painful headaches want a CT scan or an MRI. They want to find out if their headaches are caused by a serious problem, such as a brain tumour. ***But most of the time you don't need these tests.*** Here's why:

(a). ***Imaging tests rarely help.*** Doctors see many patients for headaches. *And most of them have migraine or headaches caused by tension.* Both kinds of headaches can be very painful. But a CT scan or an MRI rarely shows why the headache occurs. And they do not help you ease the pain.

(b). ***A doctor can diagnose most headaches during an office visit.*** The doctor asks you questions about your health and your symptoms. This is called a medical history. Then the doctor does a test of your reflexes, called a neurological exam. If your medical history and exam are normal, imaging tests usually will not show a serious problem.

(c.) ***CT scans have risks.*** A CT-scan of the head uses a low radiation dose. This may slightly increase the risk of harmful effects. Risks from radiation exposure may add up, so it is best to avoid unnecessary radiation. **The results of your test may also be unclear. This can lead to more tests and even treatment that you do not need.**

(d). *Imaging tests cost money*. Costs of an unnecessary scan may be higher if the results are unclear and your doctor orders more tests or treatment.

(2). ***When should you have an imaging test for headaches?*** In some cases, you might need a CT scan or an MRI. You might need one if your doctor cannot diagnose your headache based on your exam and medical history. Or you might need one if the exam finds something that is not normal.

C. <u>SM-3MM METHOD – ACUTE UPPER RESPIRATORT TRACT INFECTIONS (URTIS)</u>

If you have a fever with other common symptoms such as the coughs, nasal complaints, sore-throats, body-ache or joint pains, the 4 questions that you need to ask yourself in the SM-3MM method are as follow:

1. Do you have persistently high temperatures throughout the day and night (above 38 °C) for more than 3 days?

2. Did you just visit a waterfall, rapid, river, flooded area, pool, canal or lake? (To rule out a Leptospirosis infection)

3. Do you have abnormal bleeding from the gums, nose or noticed blood in the urine, stools or vomit?

4. Do you have jaundice (yellow skin and eyes)?

If the answers are NOES to all of the above questions, then you just need a simple treatment with the following medication:

1. Anti-Pyretic (to reduce fever) and pain relievers for fever, sore throat and headache. The most commonly used anti-pyretic and pain relievers in Malaysia is a **Paracetamol.**

2.   Anti-histamines or decongestant nasal sprays or drops. Use anti-histamines to relieve the nasal symptoms. Adults can use decongestant drops or sprays for up to five days. Prolonged use can cause rebound symptoms.

3.   Cough syrups.

4.   Drink plenty of fluids. For me plain water is the best. **The colder the water is the better, as advised by the CDC, US**. So drink water from the fridge, or iced water or you can take an ice cream. For older patients you could also take any one of the isotonic drinks, and the colder it is the better. Avoid caffeine and alcohol, which can dehydrate you.

5.   Relieve your sore-throat. Take any lozenges, a saltwater gargle or any ready-made gargles. You could also suck on ice cubes or take ice cream.

6.   Rest. If possible, stay home from work or school especially if you have a high fever or a bad cough or are drowsy after taking the medication. This will give you a chance to rest as well as reduce the chances that you will infect other people.

CHOOSING WISELY RECOMMENDATIONS FOR URTIs.

1.   **FOR DOCTORS**

     a.   ***Infectious Diseases Society of America.***

       (1)   .   *Avoid prescribing antibiotics for upper respiratory infections*. The majority of acute upper respiratory infections (URTIs) are **viral** in aetiology and ***the use of antibiotic treatment is ineffective, inappropriate and potentially harmful***.

       (2).   Symptomatic treatment for URTIs should be directed to maximize relief of the most prominent symptom(s). It is important that health care providers have a dialogue with their patients and provide education about the **consequences of misusing antibiotics in viral infections**, which may lead to increased costs, antimicrobial resistance and adverse effects.

b.   ***American Academy of Family Physicians.*** Don't routinely prescribe antibiotics for acute mild-to-moderate sinusitis unless symptoms last for ten or more days, or symptoms worsen after initial clinical improvement.

2.   **<u>FOR PATIENTS</u>**

a.   **<u>Colds, Flu, and Other Respiratory Illnesses in Adults.</u>**

(1).   ***When you need antibiotics - and when you don't.*** If you have a sore throat, cough, or sinus pain, you might expect to take antibiotics. After all, you feel bad, and you want to get better fast. ***But antibiotics don't help most respiratory infections, and they can even be harmful.*** Here's why:

(a).   Antibiotics kill bacteria, not viruses.

(b).   Antibiotics fight infections caused by bacteria. But most respiratory infections are caused by viruses. Antibiotics can't cure a virus.

(c).   Viruses cause:

    i.   All colds and flu.

    ii.   Almost all sinus infections.

    iii.   Most bronchitis (chest colds).

    iv.   Most sore throat, especially with a cough, runny nose, hoarse voice, or mouth sores.

(d).   **Antibiotics have risks**. Antibiotics can upset the body's natural balance of good and bad bacteria.

(e).   Antibiotics can cause:

    i.   Nausea, vomiting and severe diarrhoea.

    ii.   Vaginal infections.

    iii.   Nerve damage.

    iv.   Torn tendons.

v.   Life-threatening allergic reactions. Many adults go to emergency rooms because of antibiotic side effects.

(2).   ***Overuse of antibiotics is a serious problem***. Wide use of antibiotics breeds "superbugs." These are bacteria that become resistant to antibiotics. They can cause drug-resistant infections, even disability or death. The resistant bacteria (the superbugs) can also spread to family members and others.

(3).   *Overuse of antibiotics leads to high costs.* Drug-resistant infections usually need more costly drugs and extra medical care. And sometimes you need a hospital stay. In the U.S., this costs over $20 billion a year.

b.   <u>Colds, Flu, and Other Respiratory Illnesses in Children.</u>   Antibiotics for a Sore Throat, Cough, or Runny Nose, when children need them - and when they don't?

(1).   If your child has a sore throat, cough, or runny nose, you might expect the doctor to prescribe antibiotics. ***But most of the time, children don't need antibiotics to treat a respiratory illness***. In fact, antibiotics can do more harm than good. Here's why:

(a).   Antibiotics fight bacteria, not viruses.

(b).   If your child has a bacterial infection, antibiotics may help. But if your child has a virus, antibiotics will not help your child feel better or keep others from getting sick.

(c).   The Common Cold and Flu are both viruses.

(d).   Chest colds are also usually caused by viruses.

(e).   Bronchiolitis is a particular type of chest cold that often causes wheezing and can make young infants very sick. It is also caused by a virus.

(f)   Most sinus infections (sinusitis) are caused by viruses. The symptoms are a lot of mucus in the nose and post-nasal drip. ***Mucus that is coloured does not necessarily mean your child has a bacterial infection***.

(2).   Antibiotics do not help treat viruses and some infections. The flu is always caused by a virus.

(3).   Sometimes bacteria can cause sinus infections, but even then the infection usually clears up on its own in a week or so. Many common ear infections also clear up on their own without antibiotics.

(4).   ***Most sore throat are caused by viruses.*** But some sore throat, like strep throat, are bacterial infections. Symptoms include fever, redness, and trouble swallowing. Your doctor will decide if your child needs a strep test. If the test shows it is strep, then the doctor will prescribe antibiotics.

(5).   ***When does your child need antibiotics?***

    (a).   Your child MIGHT have a bacterial infection in these cases, and you should check with the doctor if these happen:

        i.   A **cough** does not get better in **14 days**.

        ii.   Symptoms of a sinus infection do not get better in 10 days, or they get better and then worse again.

        iii.   Your child has a nasal discharge and a fever of **at least 102°F (38.9°C)** for several days in a row, or nasal discharge and a headache that won't go away.

    (b)   Your child WILL need antibiotics in these cases:

        i.   If the child has a bacterial form of pneumonia.

        ii.   Whooping cough (pertussis) is diagnosed.

        iii.   Your child has strep throat, based on a rapid strep test or a throat culture.

    (c)   REMEMBER: For infants younger than 3 months of age, call your paediatrician for any fever above 100.4° F (38°C). Very young infants can have serious infections that might need antibiotics and even might need to be admitted into the hospital.

(6).   *Antibiotics have risks.* Side effects from antibiotics are a common reason that children go to the emergency room. The drugs can cause diarrhoea or vomiting, and about 5 in 100 children have allergies to them. Some of these allergic reactions can be serious and life-threatening.

(7).   *The misuse and overuse of antibiotics encourages bacteria to change,* so that medicine don't work as well to get rid of them. This is called ***"antibiotic resistance."*** When bacteria are resistant to the medicine used to treat them, it's easier for infections to spread from person to person. Antibiotic-resistant infections are also more expensive to treat and harder to cure.

(8).   When used incorrectly, antibiotics waste money. Most antibiotics do not cost a lot. But money spent on medicine that are not needed is money wasted. In severe cases, infections that are resistant to antibiotics can cost thousands of dollars to treat.

D.   <u>SM-3MM METHOD - YOUNG WOMEN WITH HIGH CHOLESTEROLS, OVARIAN CYSTS, HEART PROBLEMS AND OSTEOPOROSIS.</u>

There you are, the 3 Minutes Management for 3 different common medical problems. All three medical problems above require you to ask and answer 4 different questions to know whether you only need a simple treatment or you need a more complex treatment. I also showed that the recommendations given by the Choosing Wisely Projects were almost similar to what I advocated in this book.

I hope that you can calculate the timing from you start asking the above questions until you finish answering the questions, whether yeses or noes. I am sure that you won't take more than 3 minutes to do that as I claim. However, "time is gold". It is very precious and important, and to take 3 minutes to ask the above questions and to answer them is still a long time for me.

Therefore, for the above 4 problems in young women i.e. High Cholesterols, Ovarian Cysts, Heart Problems or Osteoporosis, you just need to ask one question instead of 4 questions. Yes, you just need to ask one question for the above 4 problems in **young women.**

For these problems, sometimes I had patients who were young ladies (below 50 years old) asking the following questions:

1. "Doctor, I had my blood tests done recently and I was found to have high blood cholesterol levels. I am on medication now. Could you repeat my blood tests and check whether I need to continue my medication?" said a 30 year old.

2. "I'm worried about having ovarian cysts. Can you refer me to a gynaecologist for an ultra-sound?" said another 25 year old.

3. "I have this chest pain off and on for the past one week. Can you do an ECG or refer me to a cardiologist?" another young lady would ask me.

4. "I am worried about having bone problems (? Osteoporosis). Can you refer me for a bone scan"? Asked another forty something lady.

For all of the above four medical problems in young women i.e. Hypercholesterolemia, Ovarian cysts, Coronary Heart Disease (CHD) and Osteoporosis, you just need to ask one question.

That one question you should ask yourself is **"Am I menopausal**?" If the answer is NO, then you don't even have to check for your blood cholesterol levels, or do an ultra-sound scan to look for ovarian cysts, or have your heart checked for a Coronary Heart Disease (CHD) or check for an Osteoporosis because they are all insignificant.

All the above four problems are not significant in young women. They will become significant when you are much older (above 50 years old) and when you are menopause. That's why we don't even check our young RMAF lady pilots (either helicopters, transport air-crafts or even our female fighter pilots) for all of the above problems.

Since whatever our RMAF aviation doctors are practising is by following whatever the Royal Air Force (RAF), UK's aviation doctors are practicing, it means that even the RAF, UK do not check their lady pilots for the above problems. If these problems are very important and significantly affecting the health of young women, then I am very sure that they would have done that a long time ago.

For the cholesterol level, if we check Malaysians, 60% to 80% of us would have high blood cholesterol levels. It is a good business then. If we check 100 normal Malaysians for the blood cholesterol levels, we could easily get 60 to 80 patients.

In young women even though you have high blood cholesterol levels, your woman's hormones i.e. the oestrogens would protect your heart. That is why it is very difficult for a young woman to have a heart attack even though she has high cholesterol levels. That is also the reason why many lady doctors that I know of do not routinely check their cholesterol levels. Oestrogens also protect your bones from having the Osteoporosis.

We do check for our pilot's blood cholesterol levels, stress tests for the Coronary Heart Disease (CHD) and an ultra-sound of the abdomen if they are more than 40 years old with the rank of Lieutenant Colonel or higher, men and women pilots. Even at 40 years old, we knew that it was still too early for these investigations to be done for women. We never do any bone density scan in the military. All of these problems were also not an issue when we checked our 'Angkasawan female candidates'.

As for the ovarian cysts, you can google for the biggest ovarian cysts in the world and you will be directed to a young lady in Mexico. (This was not the biggest, the biggest ovarian cyst was in a Vietnamese lady, which weighed 52kg). She was a 24 years old lady that lived in a rural area. When her abdomen became really big then she decided to go to the hospital. The doctors removed a 32kg ovarian cyst, which measured about half a meter in diameter. She had recovered fully after the operation.

In Malaysia, if you don't notice any obvious abdominal swelling, then you don't have to do the abdominal or pelvis ultrasound scans to look for the cysts. Most of the time if the cysts are present, they are not big enough to justify for an operation to remove them. And as I mentioned above, I have many patients that went for a routine ultra-sound scan (i.e they didn't have any signs and symptoms at all) but ended up with a major operation, for e.g. with a Total Abdominal Hysterectomy With Bilateral Salpingo-Oophorectomy (TAHBSO) operation (Total removal of the uterus, ovaries, fallopian tubes and cervix).

I know a lady medical professor who is more than 50 years old, who never had any routine abdominal or pelvis ultrasound and bone density scan done in her whole life, did not know her blood cholesterol levels and never checked her heart for a possible heart problem. And she used to be one of the top students at her university and the only foreign student that received an honours medical degree in her class.

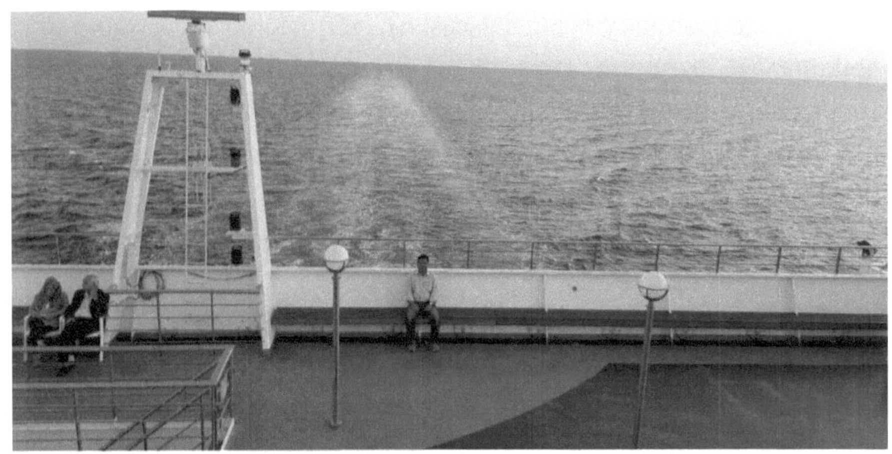

Picture-10: Crossing The Mediterranean Sea.

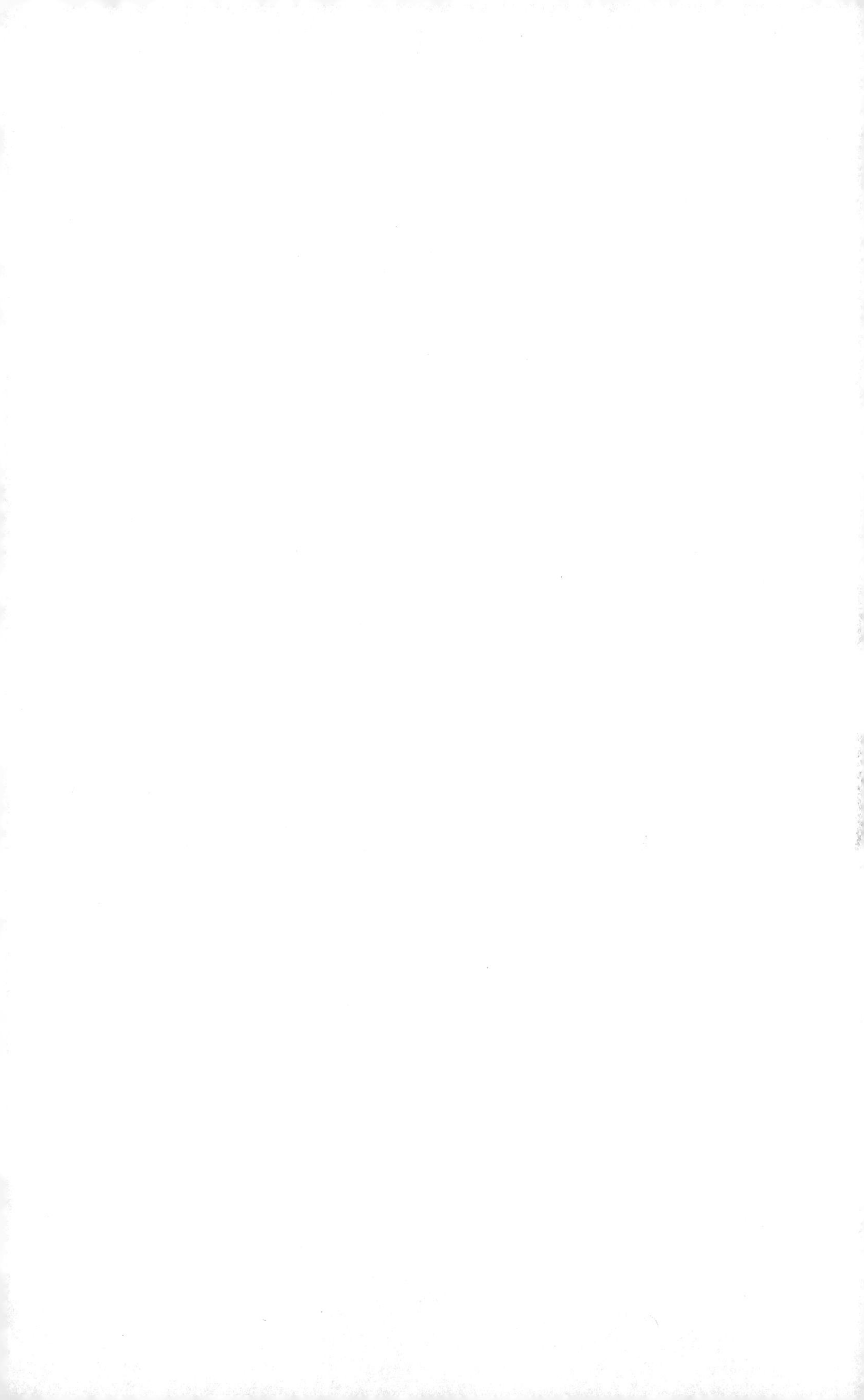

www.ingramcontent.com/pod-product-compliance
Lightning Source LLC
Chambersburg PA
CBHW031111250726
48655CB00004B/1665